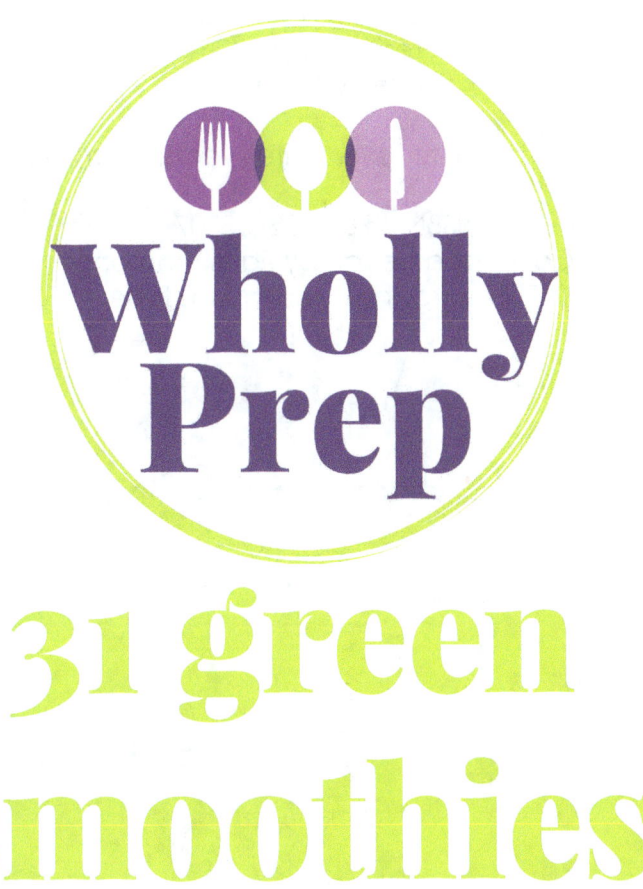

31 green smoothies

a Wholly Prep recipe book by Spirited Vegan

By Farin Montañez

Published 2018 in Fresno, CA, USA

Text and photography copyright ©2018 by Farin Montañez
All rights reserved. No part of this book may be used or reproduced in any manner whatsoever without written permission, except in the case of brief quotations embodied in critical articles or reviews.

Published by
Farin Montañez
Spirited Vegan
2814 E Brown Ave
Fresno, CA 93703
SpiritedVegan.com

Send feedback to farin.spiritedvegan@gmail.com

ISBN: 978-1732403307
Cover and design by Farin Montañez
Photography by Farin Montañez

Disclaimer: All information presented in this book is for informational purposes only. These statements have not been evaluated by the Food and Drug Administration. This book is not intended to diagnose, treat, cure or prevent any disease and is not intended to be a substitute or replacement for any medical treatment. Please seek the advice of a healthcare professional for your specific health concerns.

This book is for entertainment purposes only. The views expressed are those of the author alone and should not be taken as expert instructions or commands. The reader is responsible for their own actions. The author does not assume any responsibility or liability whatsoever on the behalf of the purchaser or reader of these materials.

Dedication

This recipe book is dedicated to my kids, Jazlyn and Isaac, who gave me their brutally honest opinions on the recipes contained in this book, and to my husband, Emmanuel, who didn't say a word as I turned our dining room into a temporary photo studio.

Acknowledgements

Thank you, friends and family who allowed me to fill your bellies with smoothie samples during the creation process, and special thanks to David for your photography expertise.

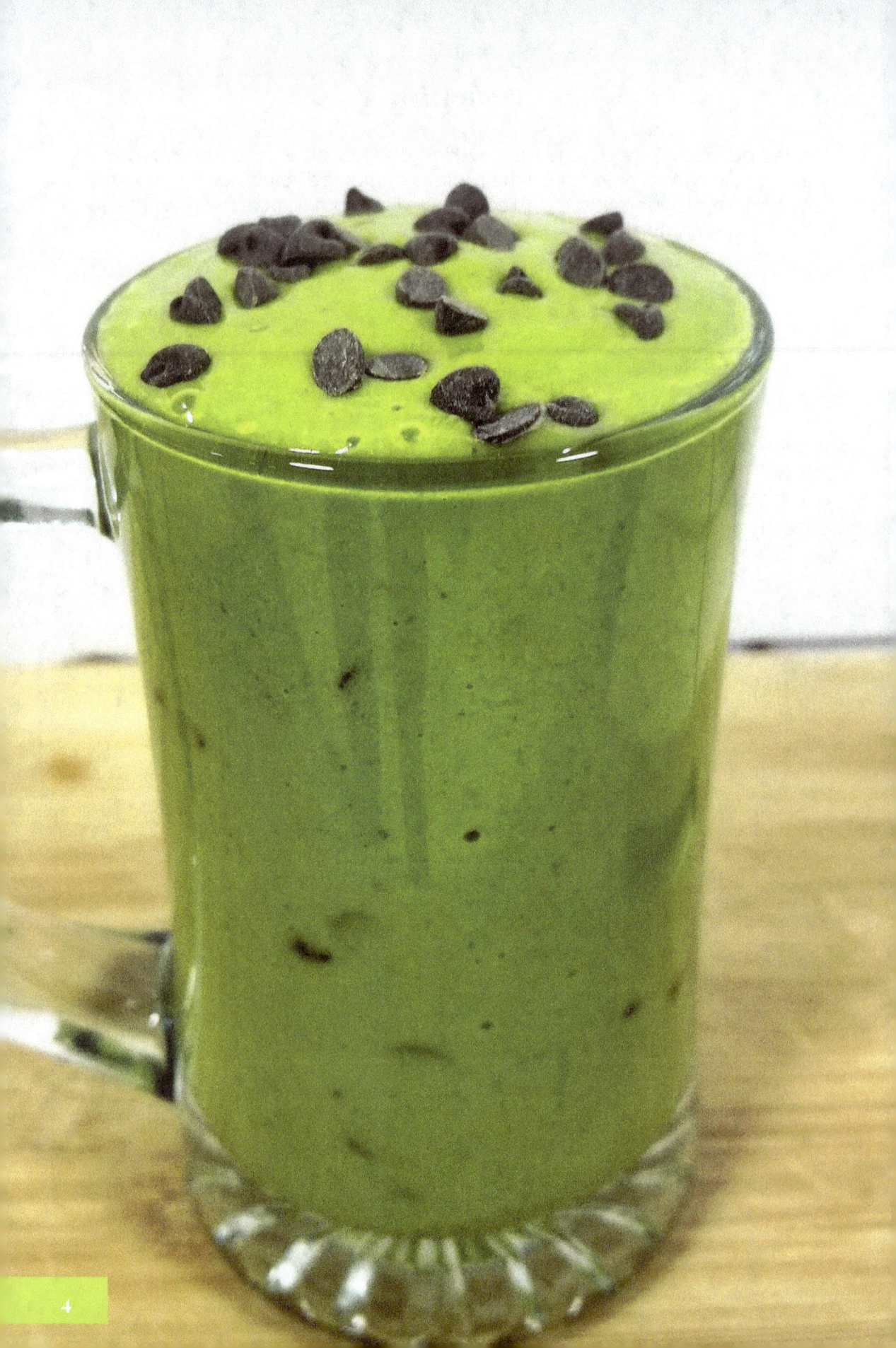

CONTENTS

Dedication 3
Acknowledgments 3
Introduction 7
   Why a Whole Food, Plant-Based Diet? 8
   What is Wholly Prep? 9

How to Use This Book 10
   Let's Talk Fruit 11
   A Word on Greens 11
   What About Equipment? 12
   Why Smoothies and Not Juice? 12

Recipes 13

Almond Strong	14
Avo-Melon	15
Beach Bum	16
Berry Banana 'N' Greens	17
Berry Vanilla	18
Creamy Cherry-Lime	19
Chilly Verde	20
Choco-Cado	21
Chocolate Covered Strawberry	22
Daring Cherry	23
Frozen Cinnamon Roll	24
Ginger-Peach	25
Grapes 'N' Greens	26
Green Creamsicle	27
Green Pb&J	28
Greeña Colada	29
Green Tea Latte	30
Hawaiian Blueberry	31
Hearty Oatmeal Smoothie	32
Kids' Favorite	33
Mint Chocolate Chip	34
Minty Watermelon	35
PB Chocolate Amor	36
Peach Mango	37
Pick-Me-Up	38
Pistachio Coconut	39
Strawberry Mango 'N' Greens	40
Superfoods	41
The Cure	42
The Zinger	43
Tropical Green Smoothie	44

References & Resources 45
   Measurements & Conversions 46
   Index 47

About the Author 48

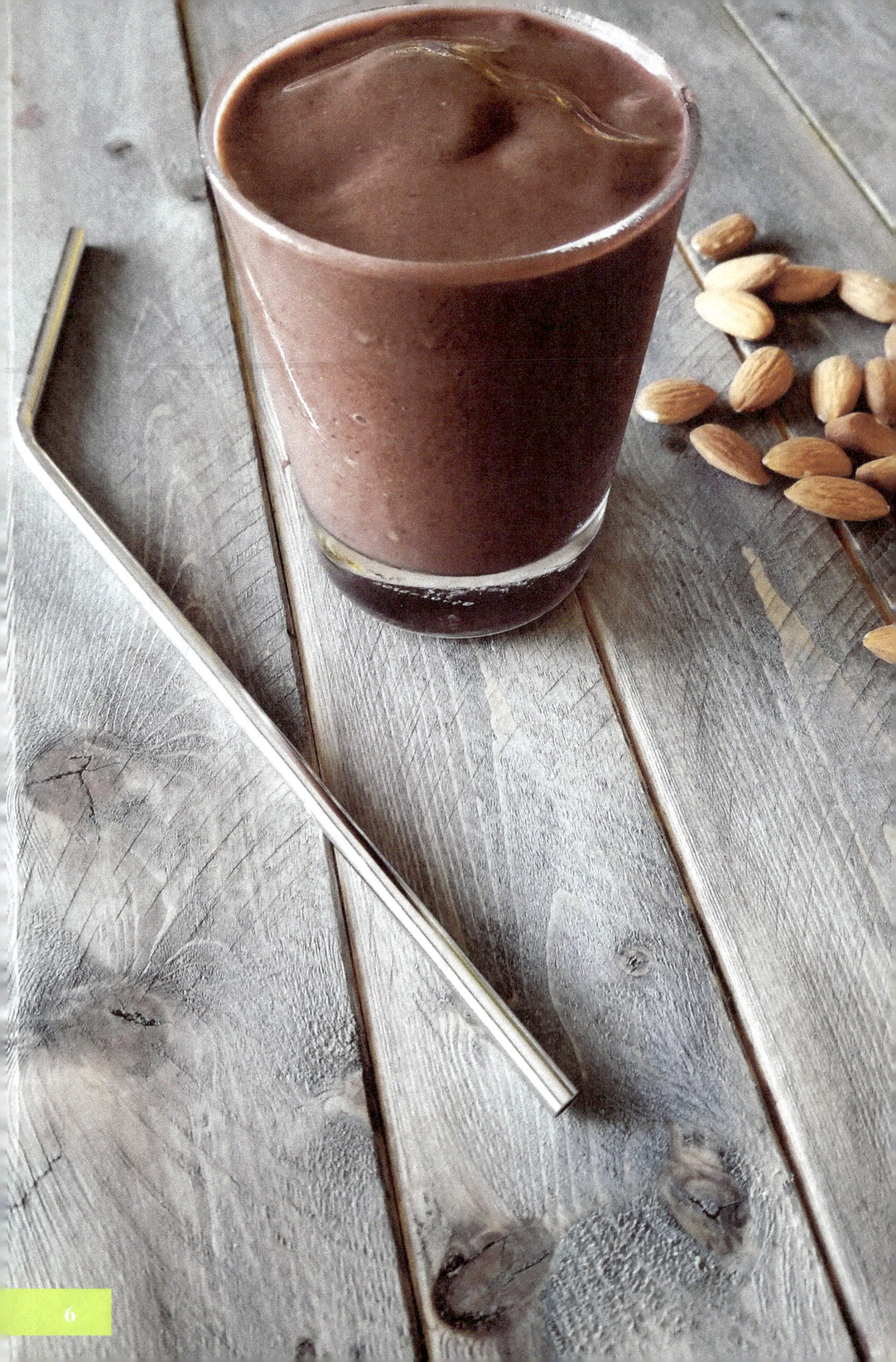

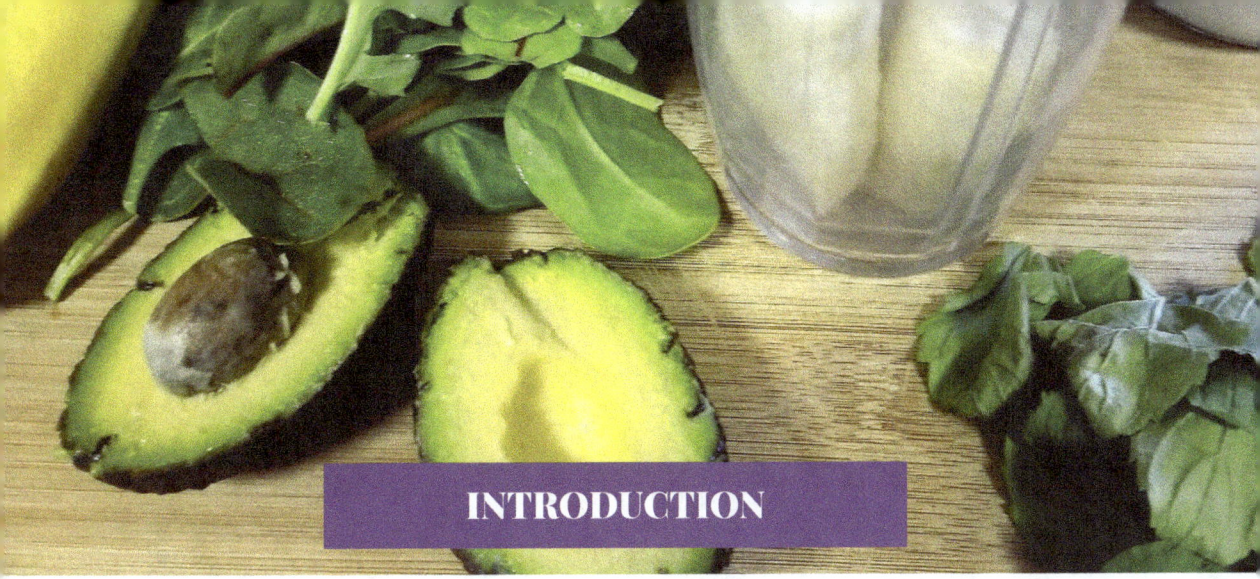

INTRODUCTION

I don't recall seeing Popeye eat a lean chicken breast before whoopin' Bluto's ass. Do you? Instead, he reached for a couple of cans of **spinach**.

Kick ass like Popeye today and every day by incorporating a green smoothie into your regimen. It's the easiest and fastest way to get a whole lot of servings of fruits and veggies in your belly and transform your health. Plus, you can take your breakfast on the go.

All of the recipes in this book fall in line with a **whole food, plant-based** diet. You might notice I never mention vegan protein powders. That's right, no powders, just whole foods! Chia, flax, and hemp seeds, along with nuts and nut butter, provide a protein boost to each smoothie. Fruits and vegetables also contain protein, along with soy and even almond milk.

These recipes were taste-tested by dozens of my closest friends. **I'll let you in on a secret:** A single smoothie could get rave reviews by a handful of testers, and the next tester would make a stink face at the first sip.

So here's the deal: **you're not going to love every smoothie in this book!** You might actually hate a few of them. And that's fine! That's why I've included a five-star rating system and space for taking notes on each page.

I challenge you to make each smoothie, one for every day of the month, and fill in the stars according to your personal taste preferences. When you've tried them all, go back and turn your 5-star favorites into your new Wholly Prep meal prepping staples.

Another Secret: There are two smoothies that literally every person loved: Chilly Verde and PB Chocolate Amor.

Oh, one more thing. These smoothies use common fruits, veggies, nuts, seeds, and liquids you can find anywhere. Seriously. There's nothing more frustrating than getting a recipe book that calls for the crushed petals of a flower found only on a specific mountain in Peru, or a super-duper-food powder that costs $73 an ounce. There's none of that crap in here. The fanciest ingredients we used are spirulina and maca — and they're optional.

Why a Whole Food, Plant-Based Diet?

The first thing that comes to mind when the word "diet" is brought up is weight loss. Why else would someone go on a diet, except to lose weight, right?

While dropping down to your body's ideal weight can be a side effect of a whole food, plant-based diet, it doesn't necessarily need to be the goal.

The best research on health, disease, and longevity shows that people who eat a diet of predominantly plant-based foods live longer and with less disease. **Plant-based diets have been shown to prevent and reverse many chronic diseases** such as heart disease and diabetes.

So the next time someone is trying to sell you on a diet that helped them lose weight, you only have to ask them one thing: has this diet been proven to prevent and reverse heart disease and diabetes and lower our risk of cancer? Then ask yourself this: **what's more important to you?** Quick weight loss, or life?

A whole food, plant-based diet is about both **adding years to your life and adding life to your years**.

What is Wholly Prep?

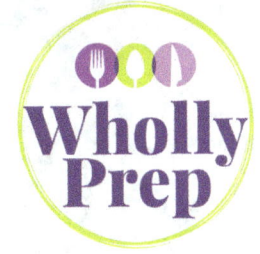

Wholly Prep is a nutritionist-created meal prepping method that helps you prepare breakfasts, lunches, and dinners for the upcoming week in about two hours.

The Wholly Prep framework is based on a philosophy of eating a **100% plant-based diet**, free from all animal products including meat, dairy, eggs, and honey. It also largely excludes processed foods, with the exception of whole grain breads and pastas, tortillas, tofu, and the like.

Wholly Prep helps you eat a wide range of leafy greens, cruciferous vegetables, starchy vegetables, non-starchy vegetables, berries, other fruits, whole grains, beans, legumes, nuts, and seeds every day.

With all of these whole plant foods in your diet, there won't be "space" for junk.

Our bodies weren't meant to consume highly processed foods, anyway. Processing food often removes fiber, concentrates calories into less bulk, and adds excessive amounts of oils, sugars, salt, and chemicals.

It's common sense that a diet rich in these processed foods would lead to obesity and chronic conditions such as heart disease, diabetes, and cancer.

Wholly Prep is a "no numbers" system. You'll meal prep breakfast, lunch, and dinner for the week without worrying about calories or even specific amounts of macronutrients (fat, carbohydrates, and protein).

Instead, Wholly Prep helps you **fill up on the healthiest, most nutrient-dense foods** first, with smaller portions of calorie-dense and minimally processed foods.

That means you'll be eating large portions of fruits and vegetables; smaller portions of whole grains, starchy vegetables, and beans; and the smallest portions of nuts, seeds, avocados, olives, dried fruit, and minimally processed foods like bread, nut milks, and tofu.

Because these nutrient-dense, high-fiber, highly satiating plant foods are generally lower in calories than animal foods and processed junk, it's actually hard to consume too many calories.

To put it simply, Spirited Vegan's Wholly Prep philosophy is this:

Eat food. Whole, plant-based food. And nothing but food.

Learn more at spiritedvegan.com/whollyprep.

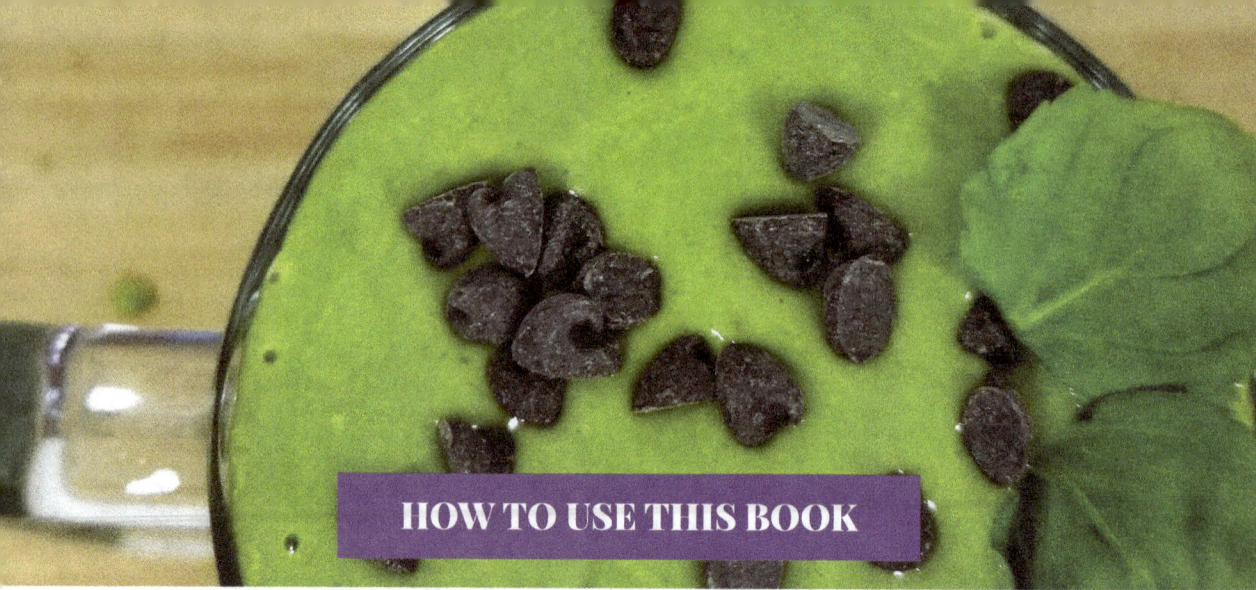

HOW TO USE THIS BOOK

31 Green Smoothies is part of the Wholly Prep framework, a system designed to help you meal prep in just two hours on the weekend — breakfast, lunch, and dinner.

Yes, you can meal prep smoothies! Each recipe has a Wholly Prep note at the bottom of the page to tell you how.

In this book, you'll find 31 tried and true green smoothie recipes to follow for a perfect start to your day or an excellent post-workout snack. That's a different smoothie every day for a month.

Each smoothie makes about a 16-ounce serving for one person, give or take a few ounces.

Use the five blank stars on each page to rate each smoothie. Then use the blank lines for notes to keep track of what you liked or disliked about the smoothie, or if you would increase or decrease the amounts of certain ingredients based on your taste and texture preferences.

Once you've tried them all, you can stick to your 5-star and 4-star favorites and use them as inspiration to create your own concoctions.

Here's the formula for the ideal whole food, plant-based green smoothie:

The Ideal Green Smoothie Formula

2-3 cups of greens. That's about two large handfuls. Aim for dark and leafy greens, such as kale, chard, collard, or spinach.
1 cup liquid. Non-dairy milk, coconut water, or just plain water.
1 to 1 ½ cups fruit. Try to incorporate a variety of colors. Eat the rainbow!
1-2 Tbsp nuts/seeds. Think chia, hemp, and flax first, and nut butter as an alternative.

Let's Talk Fruit

Fresh or frozen? Use frozen fruits when possible to achieve an optimal smoothie consistency without diluting its nutrient density by adding ice cubes. Of course, when necessary, add a few ice cubes to achieve the right consistency. Remember, **the right consistency is the one that YOU enjoy.**

Fruits are flash-frozen when ripe, so they retain their optimal nutrient content. In other words, you're going to get the same health benefits from the fruit whether you purchase it fresh or frozen.

You can also **freeze your own fresh fruit** to use later. To flash-freeze, peel and chop your fruit into bite-sized pieces, and then spread them out on a baking sheet so they're not touching each other. Freeze for an hour or two, and then place the frozen pieces in reusable freezer-safe bags. This will prevent the pieces from sticking to each other.

Fruit is a natural sweetener, so you won't need to add any sugar, artificial sweeteners, or sugary juices to your smoothies to enjoy them.

However, if your smoothie is mostly made up of veggies or less sweet fruits, toss in a couple of pitted dates to add natural sweetness and make your green smoothie more palatable.

A Word on Greens

In general, the darker the green, the more nutritious it is for your body. (That's why nutritionists love kale!)

If you don't love kale, **use greens that you like.** After all, *some* greens are better than no greens at all.

A go-to for many green smoothie enthusiasts is spinach. The cool thing about spinach is you can't even taste it in a smoothie. *(Unless you're an extremely picky 8-year-old who can detect a single leaf of any green no matter how much the other fruits and veggies mask the taste. Princess and the Pea, much?)*

Use spinach and your smoothie won't taste like a salad. It's going to taste more like a milkshake or a virgin blended drink.

Have fun experimenting! Try these greens for different tastes and textures:
- Kale
- Spinach
- Mustard greens
- Collard greens
- Rainbow chard
- Watercress
- Beet greens
- Arugula

What About Equipment?

There's no need to go out and buy a new blender. Chances are, your current blender will work just fine.

If you are in the market for a new blender, I suggest going one or two steps above the cheapest model.

I use a Nutri Ninja with Auto IQ blender because, frankly, I haven't splurged on a high-powered blender like a Vitamix or Blendtec.

The Nutri Ninja is affordable, reliable, and has pre-programmed Blend, Ultra Blend, and Smoothies settings that save time and brain power. I just push one of the pre-sets and use that 60 seconds to clean up and grab my metal straw while the Nutri Ninja does its thing.

Most people drink smoothies with straws. Please help save the world by banishing plastic straws from your home. You can buy a pack of wide stainless steel straws including a straw cleaner for cheap on Amazon, at Walmart, and several other retailers. They're reusable, easy to clean, last forever, and won't end up filling our oceans and landfills with unnecessary plastic.

Why Smoothies and Not Juice?

Fruits and veggies are perfectly packaged to deliver their nutrients, vitamins, and fiber in nature's intended way. When we juice them, we are stripping away the fiber and getting a highly concentrated dose of fructose.

Yes, we're getting some micronutrients too, but stripping the fiber from the produce and only consuming its juice causes a spike in blood sugar, triggering the body to release a large amount of insulin within the first hour of juice consumption. That spike is then followed by a crash, as the body realizes it has overdone it on the insulin. This is called rebound hypoglycemia, which can cause a person to experience varying degrees of fatigue, fainting, shakiness, nausea, confusion, headache, anxiety, and irritability. Not good!

Consuming fruits and veggies whole is the healthiest way to get your nutrients, antioxidants and, of course, fiber, but smoothies are the next-best way. Pureeing the entire fruit or vegetable is essentially like starting the digestive process by doing the "chewing" for you. Blending retains the nutrients and fiber, but just makes it easier and faster to consume your produce on-the-go.

Green smoothies are a great way to get 3 or more servings of fruits and vegetables right at the start of your day (or post-workout, or at night as dessert, or whenever the heck you want to drink one!)

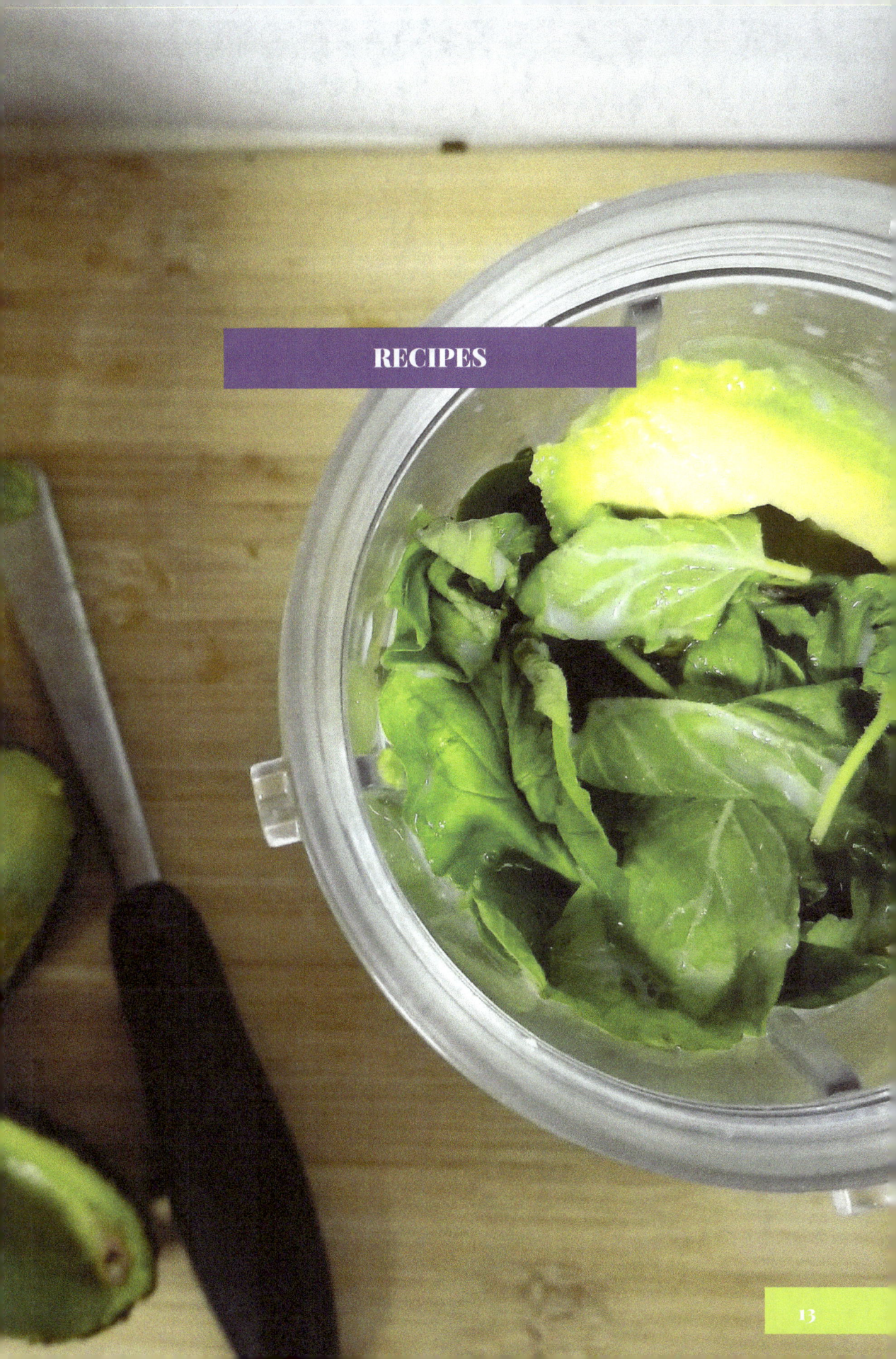

RECIPES

ALMOND STRONG

☆☆☆☆☆

INGREDIENTS

2 handfuls greens
1 cup soy milk
1 Tbsp almond butter
1 pear, sliced
1 Tbsp hemp seeds
1 frozen banana

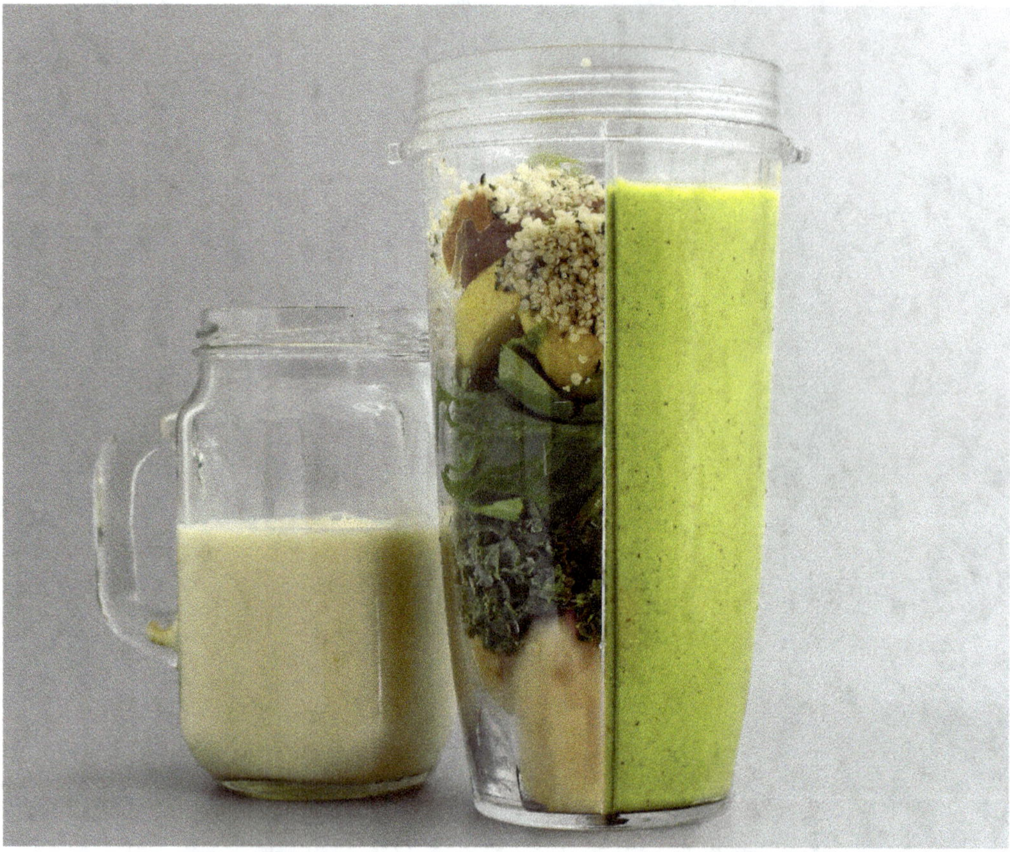

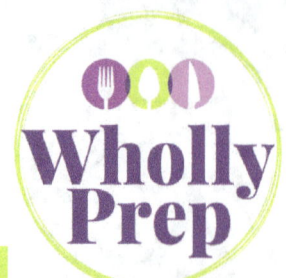

Place **greens**, **almond butter**, sliced **pear**, **hemp seeds**, and peeled, sliced **banana** in a freezer-safe container and freeze for up to 3 months.

To prepare smoothie, dump all frozen ingredients into a blender, add **soy milk**, and puree until smooth.

AVO-MELON

INGREDIENTS

2 handfuls greens
1 frozen banana
1 avocado
1 cup cantaloupe or honeydew
1 tsp hemp seeds
2 dates, pitted
1 cup water

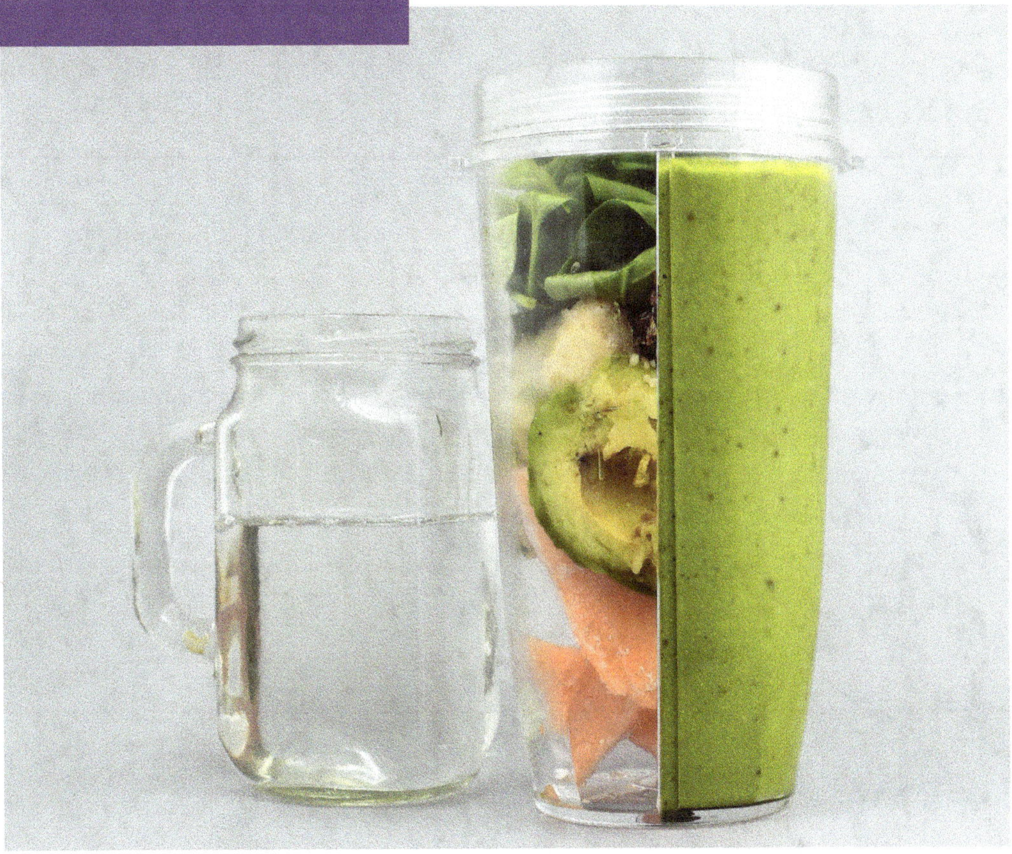

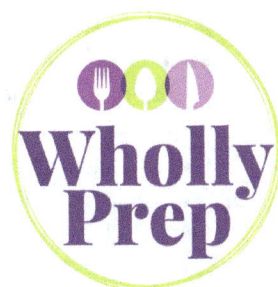

Place **greens**, peeled and sliced **banana**, **avocado**, **hemp seeds**, pitted **dates** and **melon** in a freezer-safe container and freeze for up to 3 months.

To prepare smoothie, dump all frozen ingredients into a blender, add **water**, and puree until smooth.

BEACH BUM

☆☆☆☆☆

INGREDIENTS

2 handfuls greens
1 cup coconut milk
3 mandarins
1 frozen banana
1 Tbsp chia seeds

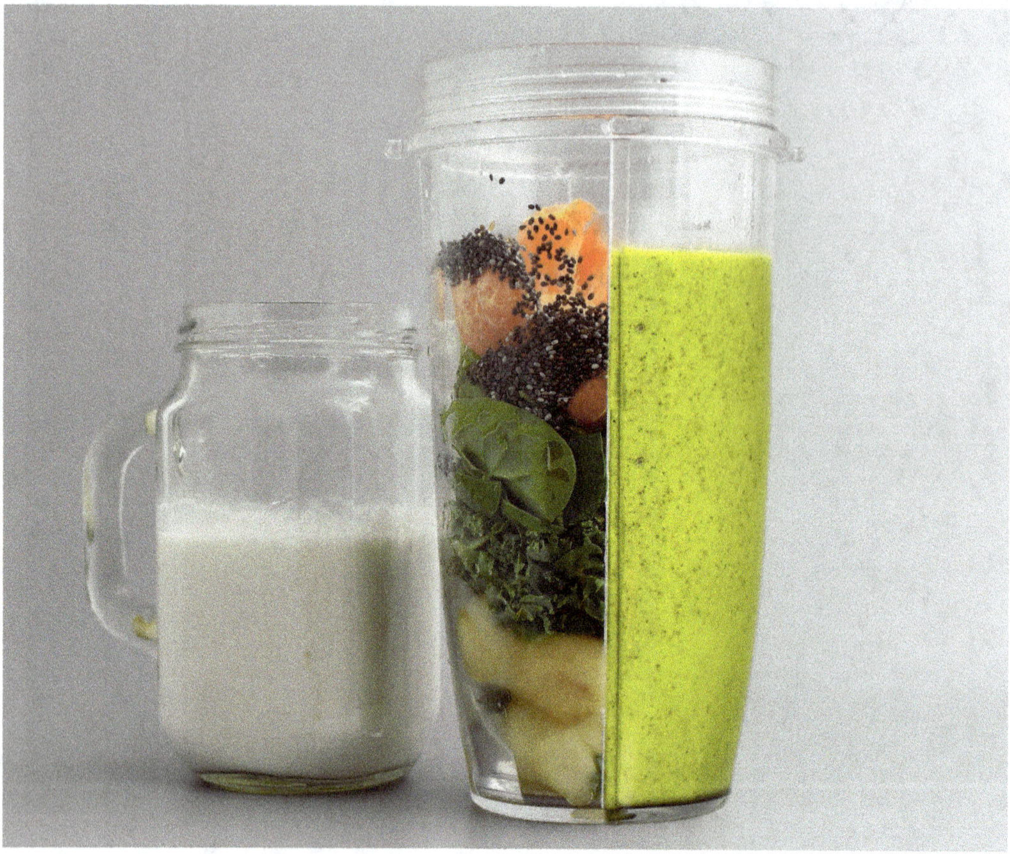

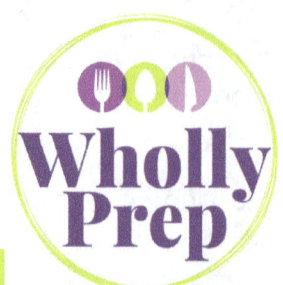

Place **greens**, peeled and sliced **banana**, peeled **mandarins**, and **chia seeds** in a freezer-safe container and freeze for up to 3 months.

To prepare smoothie, dump all frozen ingredients into a blender, add **coconut milk,** and puree until smooth.

BERRY BANANA 'N' GREENS

INGREDIENTS

2 handfuls greens
1 Tbs peanut butter
1 Tbsp flaxseed meal
1 cup frozen mixed berries
1 frozen banana
1 cup soy milk

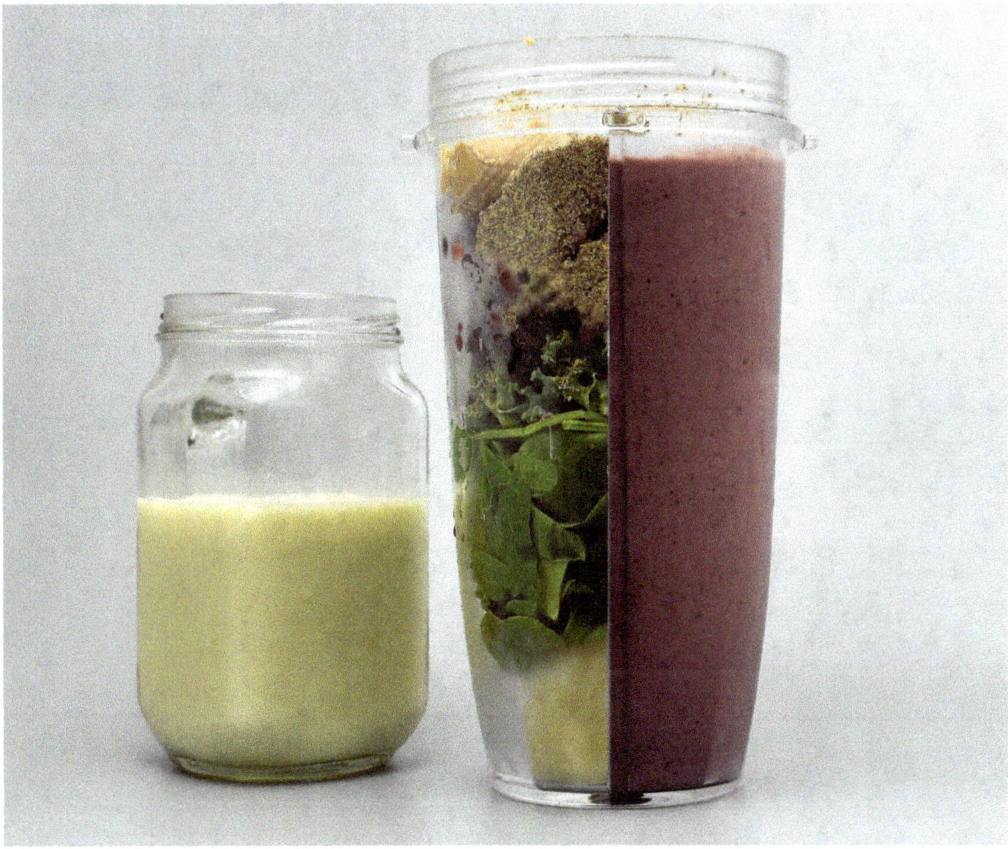

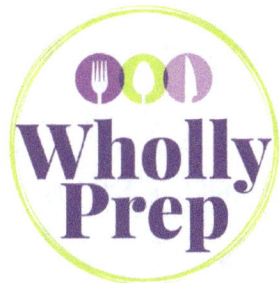

Place **greens, peanut butter, flaxseed meal, mixed berries,** and peeled, sliced **banana** in a freezer-safe bag and freeze up to 3 months.

To prepare smoothie, dump all frozen ingredients into a blender, add **soy milk,** and puree until smooth.

BERRY VANILLA

INGREDIENTS

2 handfuls greens
1 cup frozen mixed berries (raspberries, blackberries, blueberries)
½ cup frozen strawberries
1 cup vanilla almond milk (or 1 cup almond milk and 1 tsp vanilla)
1 Tbsp chia seeds
1-2 dates, pitted

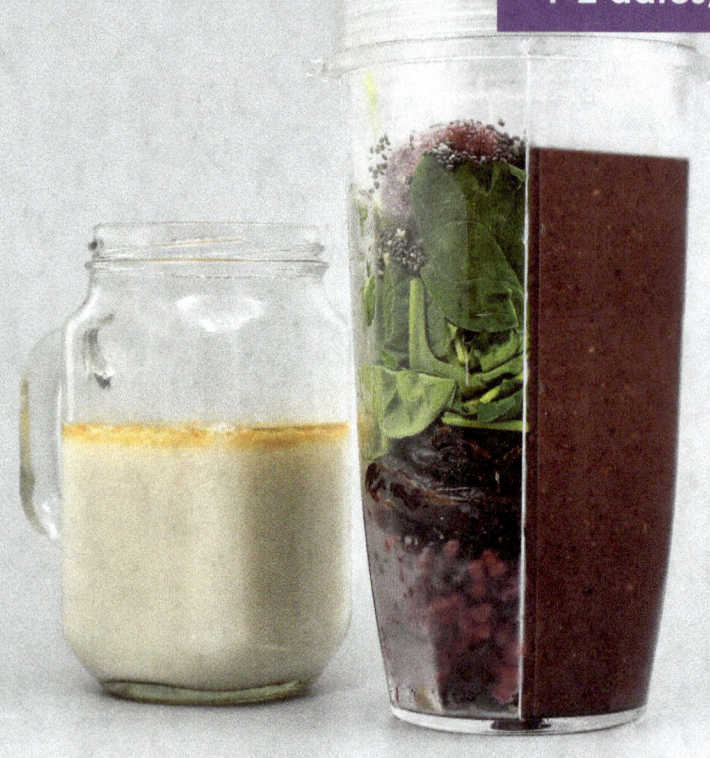

Place **greens**, pitted **dates**, **chia seeds**, and **berries** in a freezer-safe container and freeze up to 3 months.

To prepare smoothie, dump all frozen ingredients into a blender, add **almond milk** and **vanilla,** and puree until smooth.

CREAMY CHERRY-LIME

INGREDIENTS

2 handfuls greens
1 cup frozen cherries, pitted
½ cup frozen peaches
1 Tbsp chia seeds
1 cup non-dairy milk
1 Tbsp lime juice

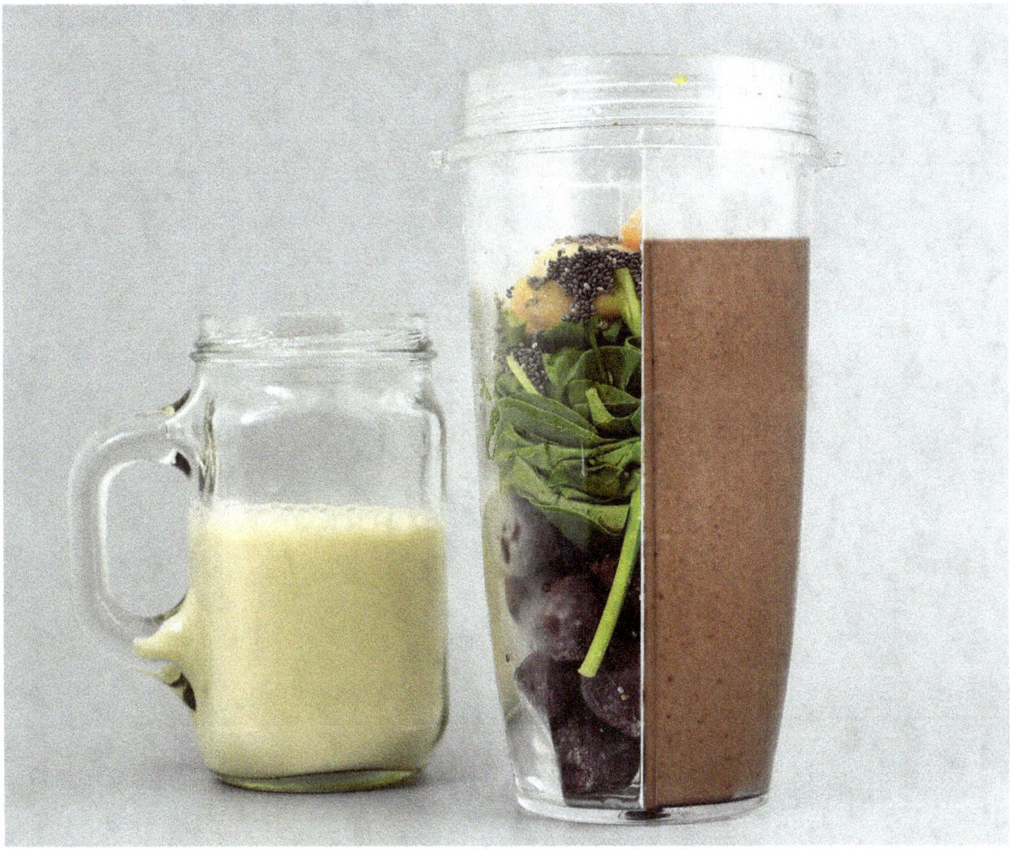

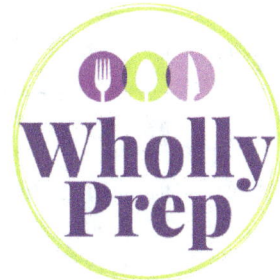

Place **greens**, pitted **cherries**, **chia seeds**, and sliced **peaches** in a freezer-safe container and freeze up to 3 months.

To prepare smoothie, dump all frozen ingredients into a blender, add **non-dairy milk** and **lime juice**, and puree until smooth.

CHILLY VERDE

INGREDIENTS

2 handfuls greens
Half a cucumber
Half a jalapeño, seeded
10 mint leaves
10 cilantro leaves
Half a lime
1/2 cup coconut water
1 handful ice

Wholly Prep

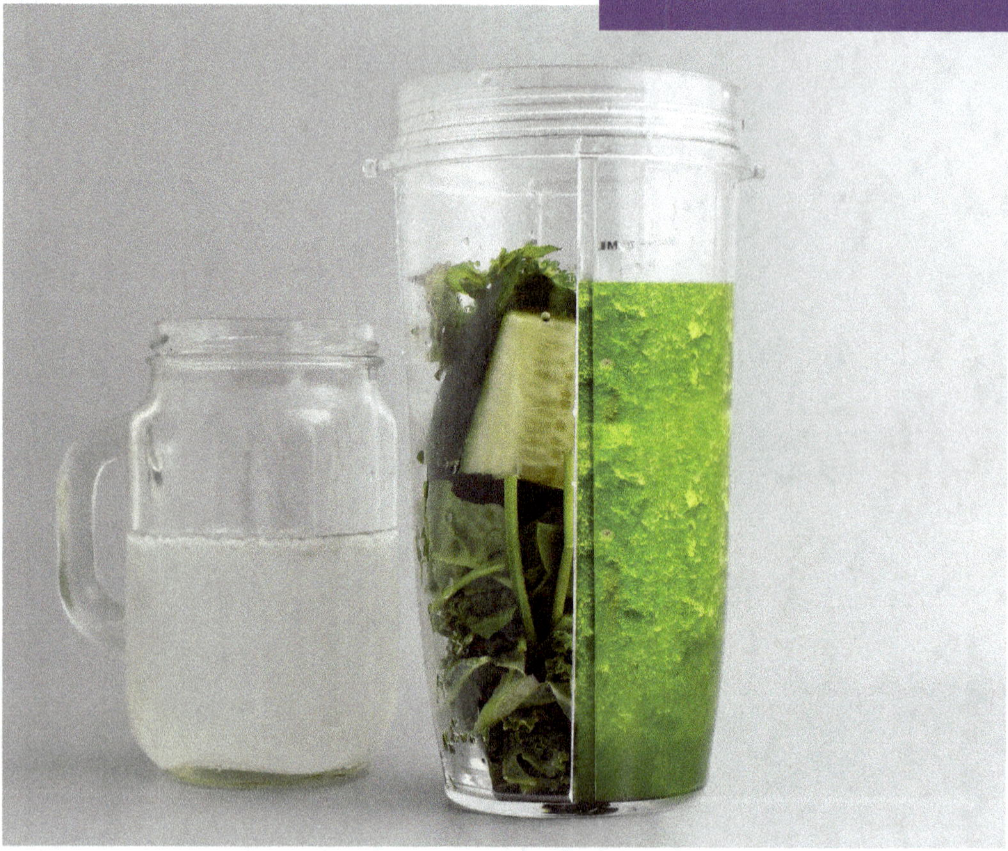

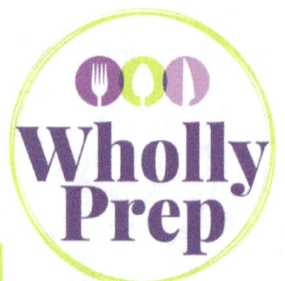

Place **greens**, **cucumber**, seeded **jalapeño**, **mint**, **cilantro**, and **lime** in a freezer-safe container and freeze up to 3 months.

To prepare smoothie, dump all frozen ingredients into a blender, add **coconut water** and **ice,** and puree until smooth.

CHOCO-CADO

INGREDIENTS

2 handfuls greens
1 frozen banana
1 avocado, pitted
3 dates, pitted
2 Tbsp cocoa powder
2 Tbsp almond butter
1 Tbsp chia seeds
1 cup almond milk
½ tsp vanilla

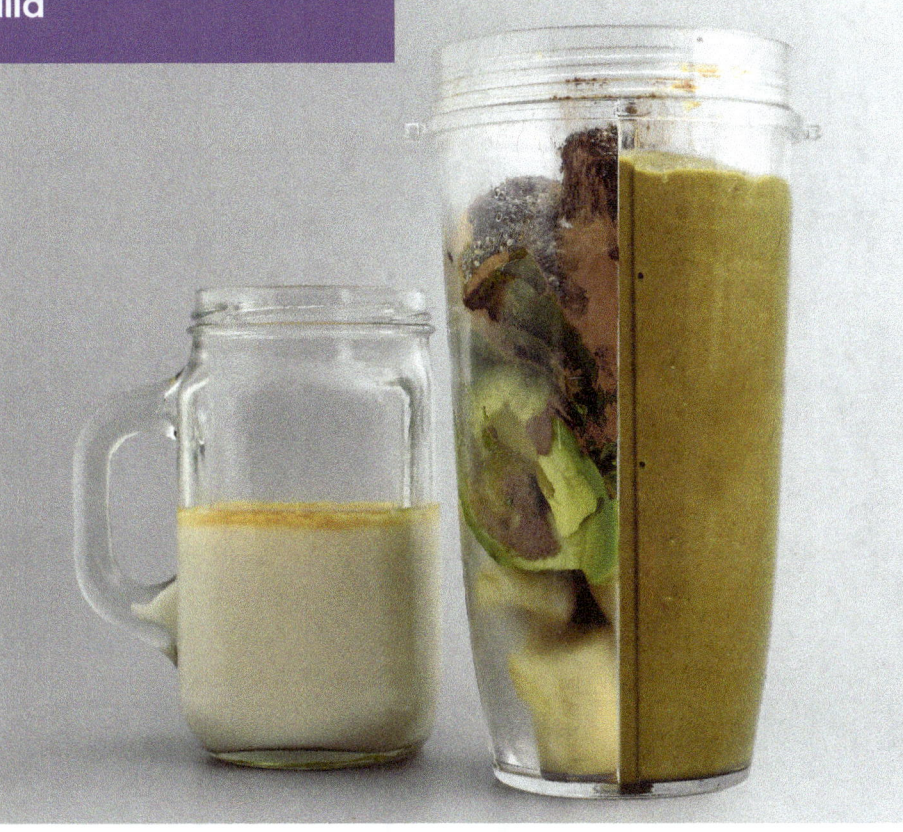

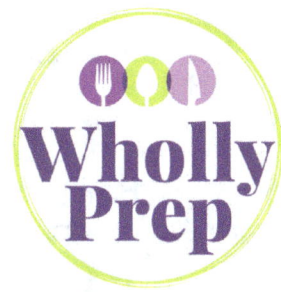

Place **greens**, pitted **avocado** and **dates**, **chia seeds**, **cocoa powder**, **almond butter**, and peeled, sliced **banana** in a freezer-safe container and freeze up to 3 months.

To prepare smoothie, dump all frozen ingredients into a blender, add **almond milk** and **vanilla**, and puree until smooth.

CHOCOLATE COVERED STRAWBERRY

INGREDIENTS

2 handfuls greens
1 cup frozen strawberries
1 avocado
1 cup non-dairy milk
1 Tbsp cocoa powder
½ tsp vanilla
2 dates, pitted

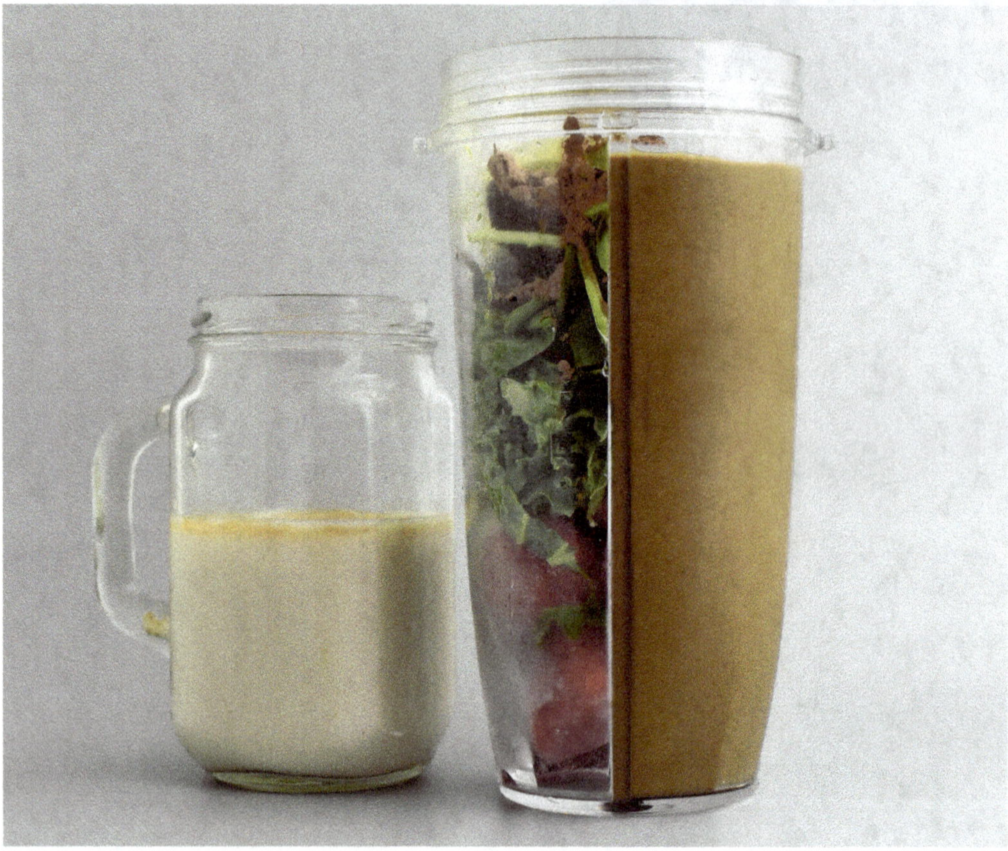

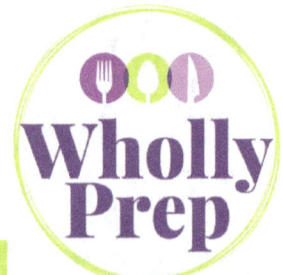

Place **greens**, pitted **avocado** and **dates**, **strawberries**, and **cocoa powder** in a freezer-safe container and freeze up to 3 months.

To prepare smoothie, dump all frozen ingredients into a blender, add **non-dairy milk** and **vanilla,** and puree until smooth.

DARING CHERRY

☆☆☆☆☆

INGREDIENTS

2 handfuls spinach
1 cup almond milk
1 cup cherries, pitted (frozen, if possible)
2 Tbsp whole almonds
½ tsp vanilla extract
½ tsp almond extract
1 date, pitted
1 handful ice, if desired

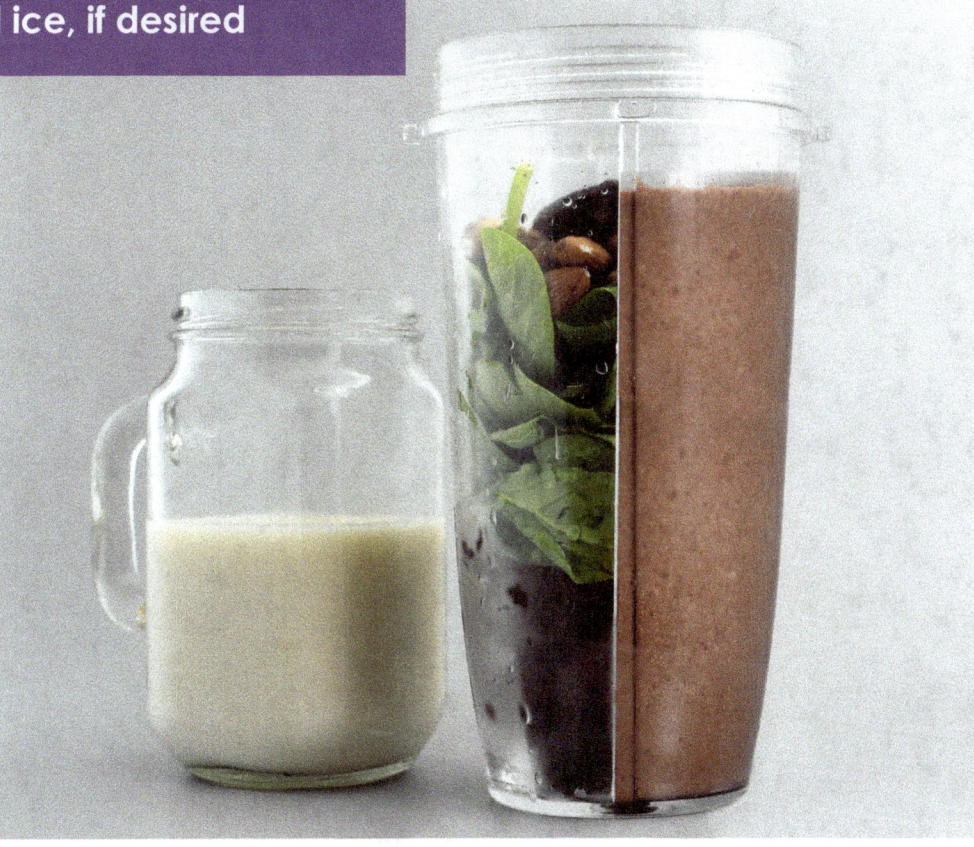

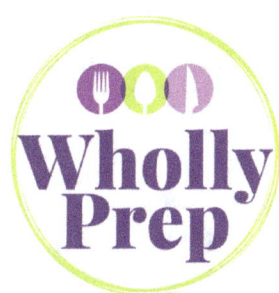

Place **spinach**, pitted **cherries** and **date**, and **almonds** in a freezer-safe container and freeze up to 3 months.

To prepare smoothie, dump all frozen ingredients into a blender, add **almond milk**, **vanilla**, **almond extract**, and **ice**, and puree until smooth.

FROZEN CINNAMON ROLL

INGREDIENTS

2 handfuls spinach
1 cup non-dairy milk
½ cup old fashioned oats
1 tsp cinnamon
½ tsp vanilla
1 frozen banana
1 Tbsp flaxseed meal
2 dates, pitted

Wholly Prep

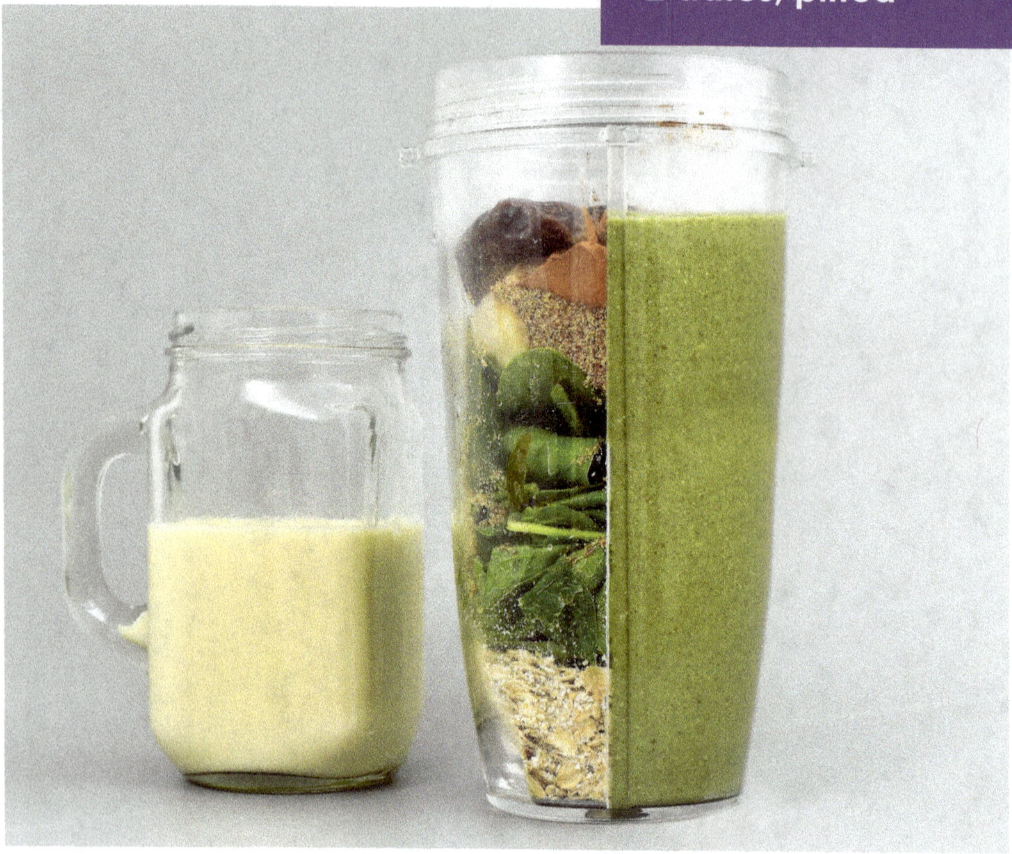

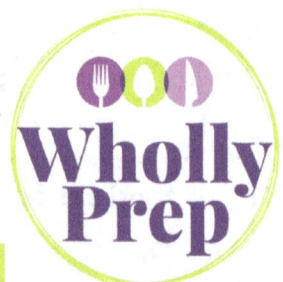

Place **spinach,** pitted **dates, flaxseed meal, cinnamon, oats**, and peeled, sliced **banana** in a freezer-safe container and freeze up to 3 months.

To prepare smoothie, dump all frozen ingredients into a blender, add **non-dairy milk** and **vanilla,** and puree until smooth.

GINGER-PEACH

INGREDIENTS

2 handfuls spinach
1 cup frozen peaches
1 cup water or coconut water
½ inch peeled ginger
1 date, pitted

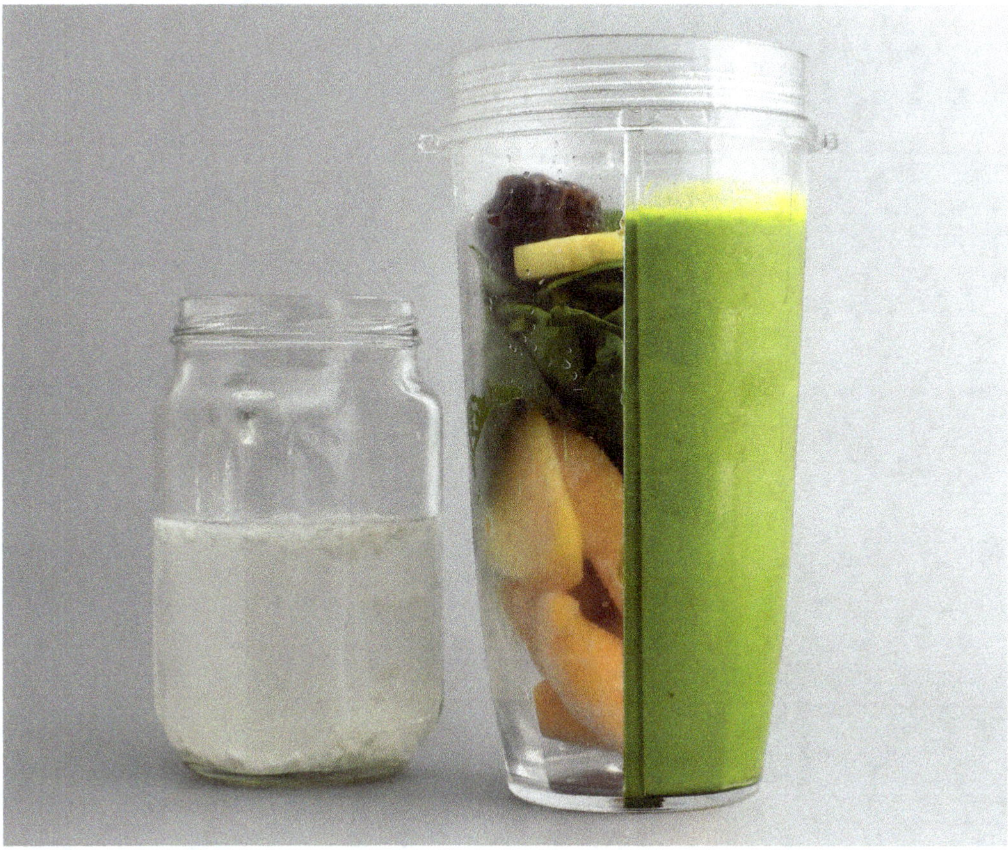

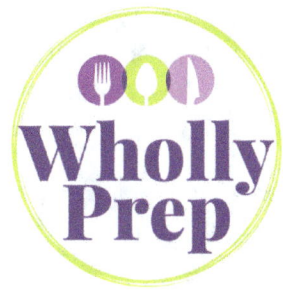

Place **spinach**, **peaches**, pitted **date** and peeled **ginger** in a freezer-safe container and freeze up to 3 months.

To prepare smoothie, dump all frozen ingredients into a blender, add **water** or **coconut water**, and puree until smooth.

GRAPES 'N' GREENS

INGREDIENTS

1 cup kale
1 medium cucumber, sliced
1 cup frozen seedless grapes
3/4 cup coconut water
6-8 inches celery
1 frozen kiwi, peeled

Wholly Prep

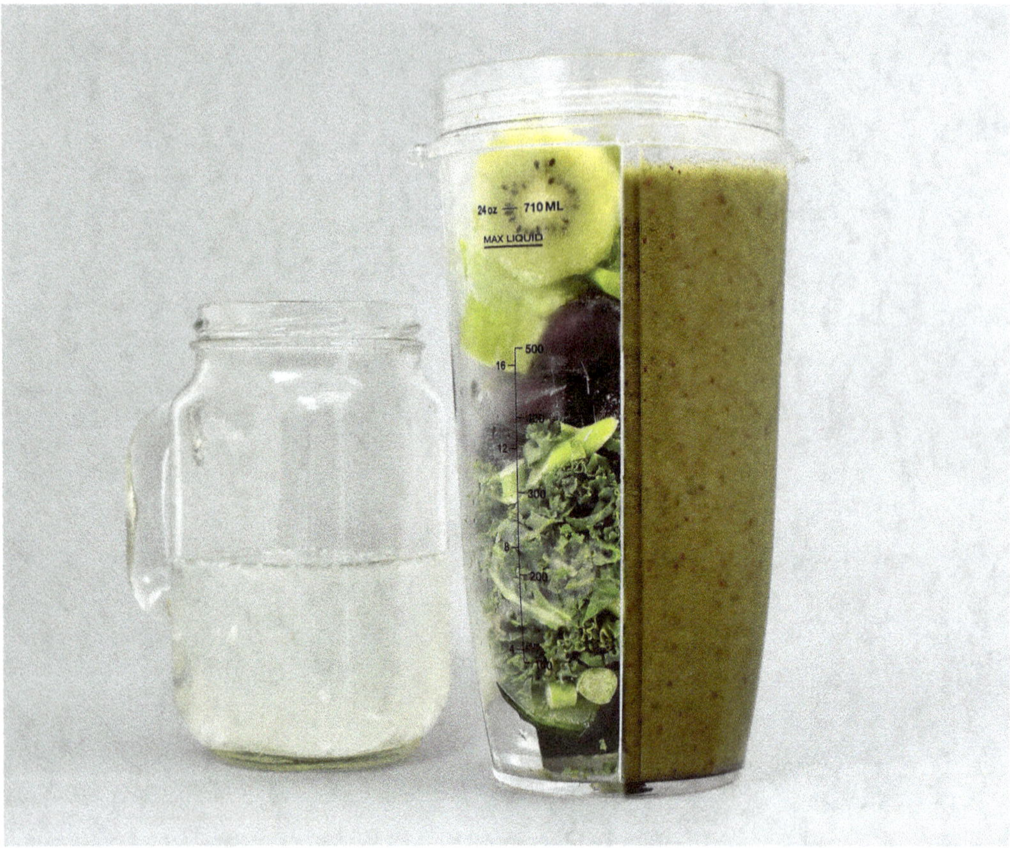

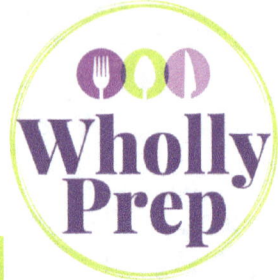

Place **kale**, sliced **cucumber, celery**, peeled **kiwi**, and **grapes** in a freezer-safe container and freeze up to 3 months.

To prepare smoothie, dump all frozen ingredients into a blender, add **coconut water,** and puree until smooth.

GREEN CREAMSICLE

INGREDIENTS

2 handfuls spinach
1 frozen banana
2 tsp vanilla extract
1 large navel orange, peeled and seeded
1 cup almond or soy milk
2 tsp orange zest

Tip: Zest the orange first, then peel and pick the seeds out of each slice. Remove as much of the pith as possible, or the smoothie will taste bitter.

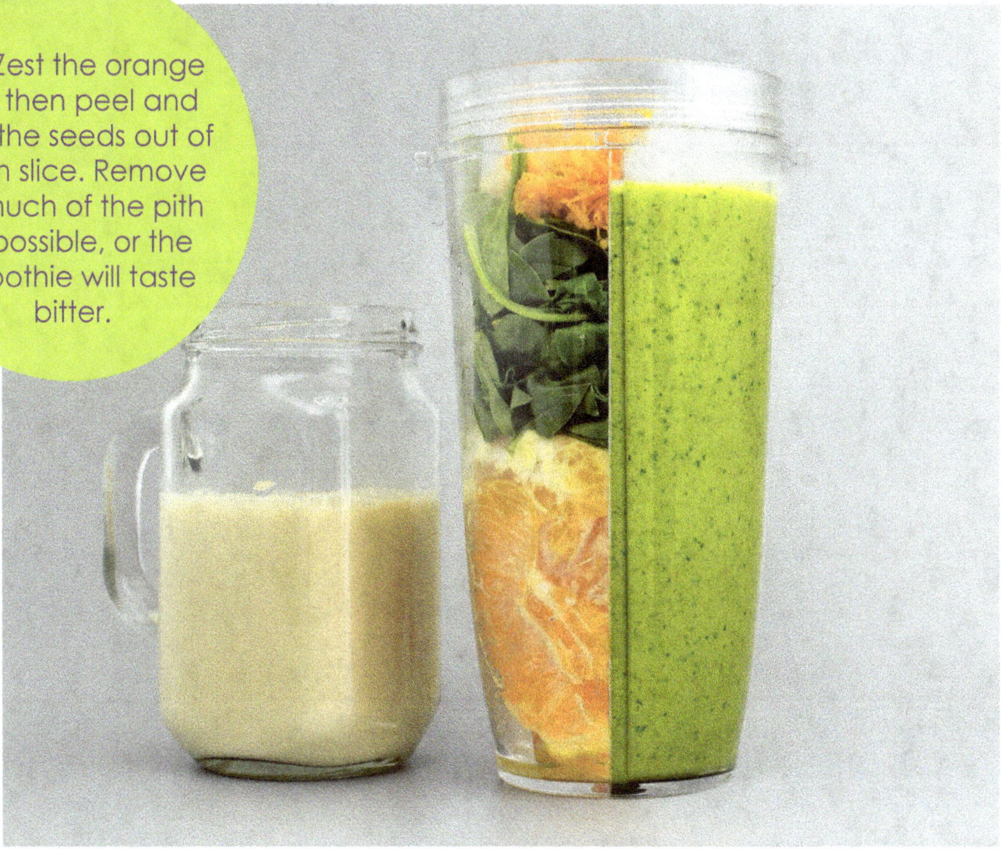

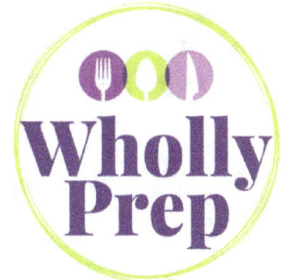

Place **spinach**, **orange zest**, peeled and seeded **orange**, and peeled, sliced **banana** in a freezer-safe container and freeze up to 3 months.

To prepare smoothie, dump all frozen ingredients into a blender, add **non-dairy milk** and **vanilla,** and puree until smooth.

GREEN PB&J

INGREDIENTS

2 handfuls of spinach
1 frozen banana
¾ cup frozen strawberries
2 dates, pitted
2 Tbsp peanut butter
¼ cup old-fashioned oats
1 cup almond milk

Wholly Prep

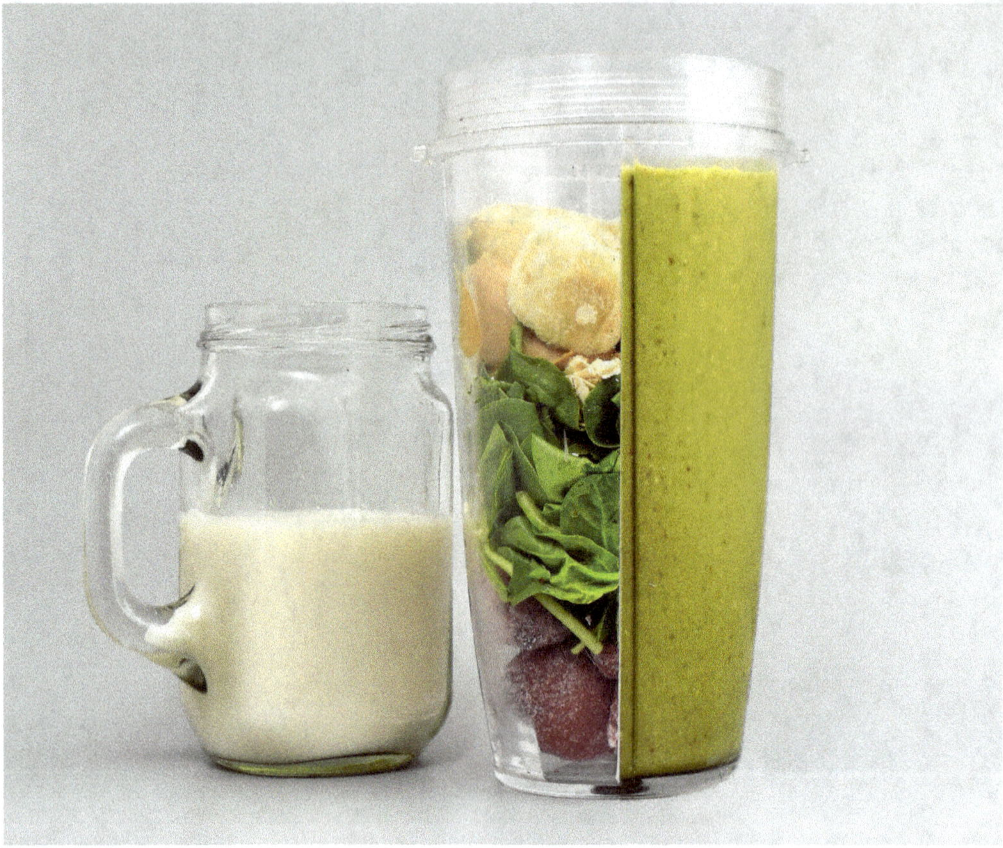

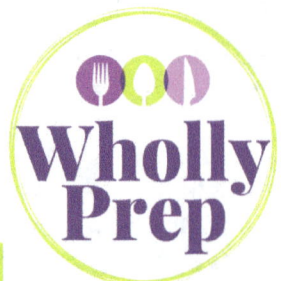

Place **spinach**, pitted **dates**, **oats**, **strawberries**, **peanut butter**, and peeled, sliced **banana** in a freezer-safe container and freeze up to 3 months.

To prepare smoothie, dump all frozen ingredients into a blender, add **almond milk,** and puree until smooth.

GREEÑA COLADA

INGREDIENTS

2 handfuls of greens
1 cup frozen pineapple chunks
1 cup coconut milk
2 Tbsp coconut flakes
½ frozen banana

Tip: Blend the coconut flakes in or garnish with them, depending on texture preferences. Use canned coconut milk for richer flavor.

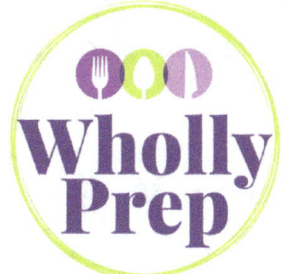

Place **greens**, **pineapple chunks**, **coconut flakes**, and peeled, sliced **banana** in a freezer-safe container and freeze up to 3 months.

To prepare smoothie, dump all frozen ingredients into a blender, add **coconut milk** and puree until smooth.

GREEN TEA LATTE

☆☆☆☆☆

INGREDIENTS

2 handfuls greens
2 frozen bananas
½ cup green tea concentrate
½ cup non-dairy milk
1 Tbsp flaxseed meal

Tip: TAZO Green Tea Latte Concentrate was used for this photo.

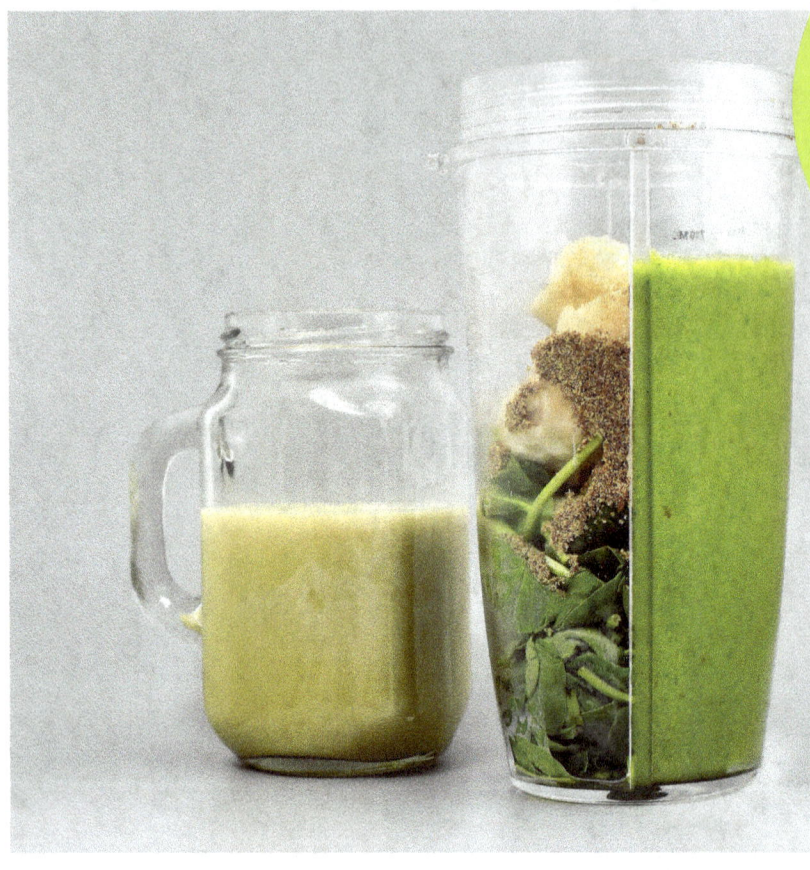

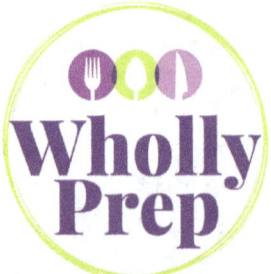

Place **greens**, **flaxseed meal**, and peeled, sliced **bananas** in a freezer-safe container and freeze up to 3 months.

To prepare smoothie, dump all frozen ingredients into a blender, add **non-dairy milk** and **green tea latte concentrate**, and puree until smooth.

HAWAIIAN BLUEBERRY

INGREDIENTS

2 handfuls greens
½ cup frozen pineapple chunks
1 orange, peeled and seeded
½ cup frozen blueberries
1 Tbsp chia seeds
¾ cup water

Wholly Prep

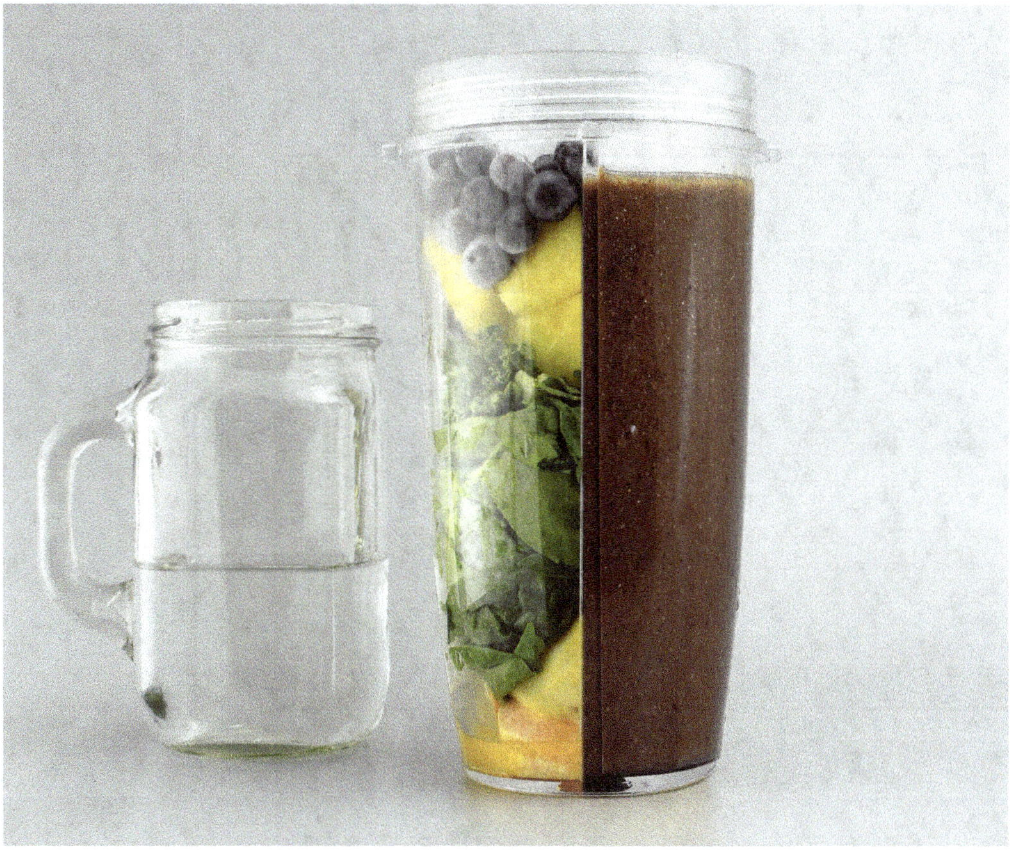

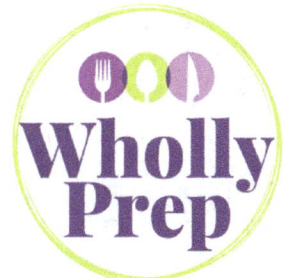

Place **greens**, **pineapple chunks**, **chia seeds**, **blueberries**, and peeled, seeded **orange** in a freezer-safe container and freeze up to 3 months.

To prepare smoothie, dump all frozen ingredients into a blender, add **water,** and puree until smooth.

HEARTY OATMEAL SMOOTHIE

☆☆☆☆☆

INGREDIENTS

2 handfuls greens
½ cup old-fashioned oats
½ cup frozen peaches
1 frozen banana
2 dates, pitted
1 cup non-dairy milk

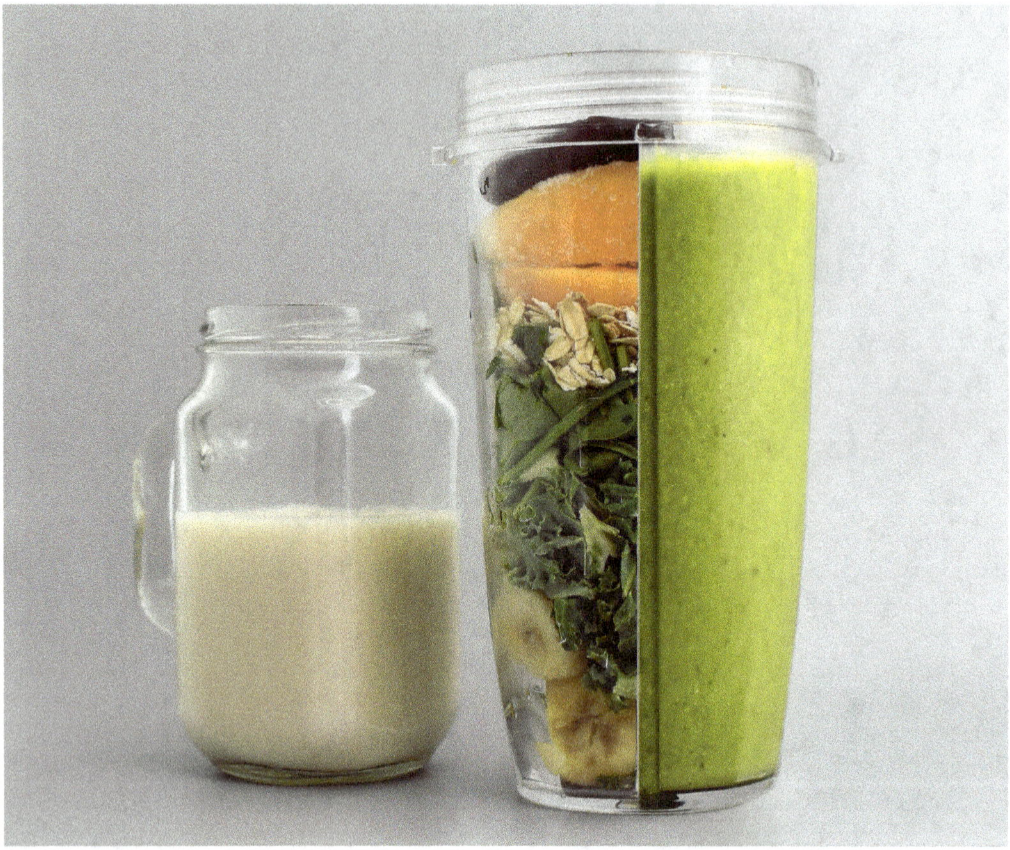

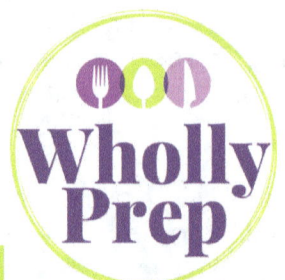

Place **greens**, pitted **dates**, **oats**, **peaches**, and peeled, sliced **banana** in a freezer-safe container and freeze up to 3 months.

To prepare smoothie, dump all frozen ingredients into a blender, add **non-dairy milk,** and puree until smooth.

KIDS' FAVORITE

INGREDIENTS

1 handful spinach
1 cup frozen strawberries
1 frozen banana
1 green apple, cored and chopped
1 Tbsp flaxseed meal
1 date, pitted
1 cup water

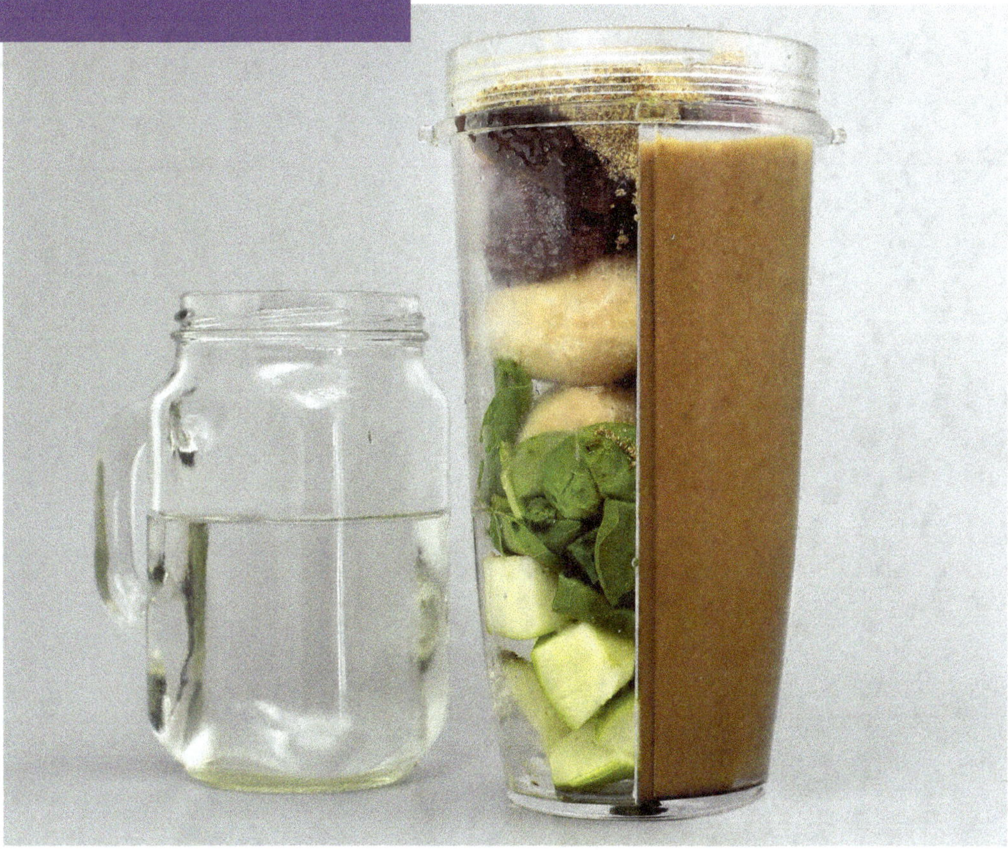

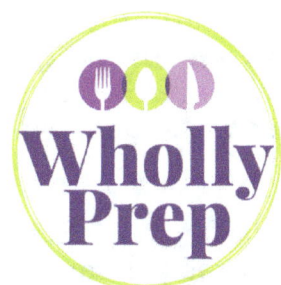

Place **spinach**, pitted **date**, **flaxseed meal**, **green apple chunks**, **strawberries**, and peeled, sliced **banana** in a freezer-safe container and freeze up to 3 months.

To prepare smoothie, dump all frozen ingredients into a blender, add **water,** and puree until smooth.

MINT CHOCOLATE CHIP

INGREDIENTS

2 handfuls greens
20-30 mint leaves
1 cup almond milk
1 avocado
1 frozen banana
1 Tbsp hemp seeds
1 Tbsp cacao nibs or mini vegan chocolate chips

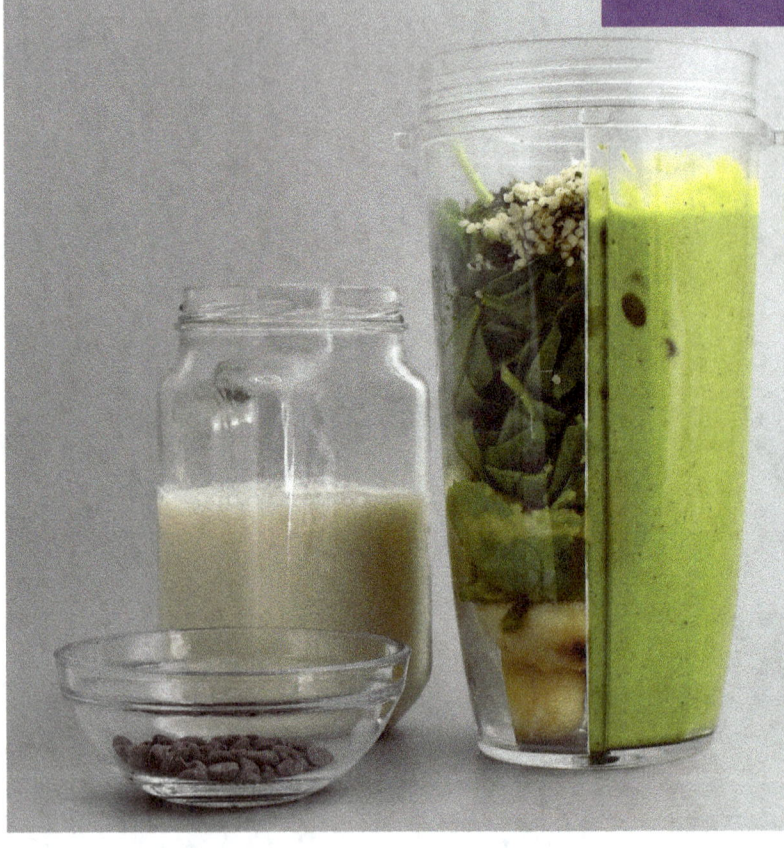

Tip: Blend the cacao nibs/chocolate chips in the smoothie or garnish with them, depending on texture preferences.

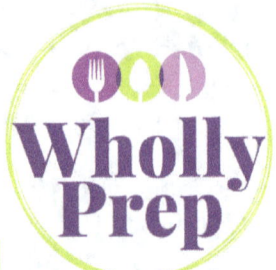

Place **greens**, pitted **avocado**, **hemp seeds**, **mint**, **cacao nibs or chocolate chips**, and peeled, sliced **banana** in a freezer-safe container and freeze up to 3 months.

To prepare smoothie, dump all frozen ingredients into a blender, add **almond milk,** and puree until smooth.

MINTY WATERMELON

INGREDIENTS

2 handfuls greens
1 1/2 cups frozen watermelon
8-10 mint leaves (about one sprig)
1/3 cup water
1 tsp lemon juice or lime juice

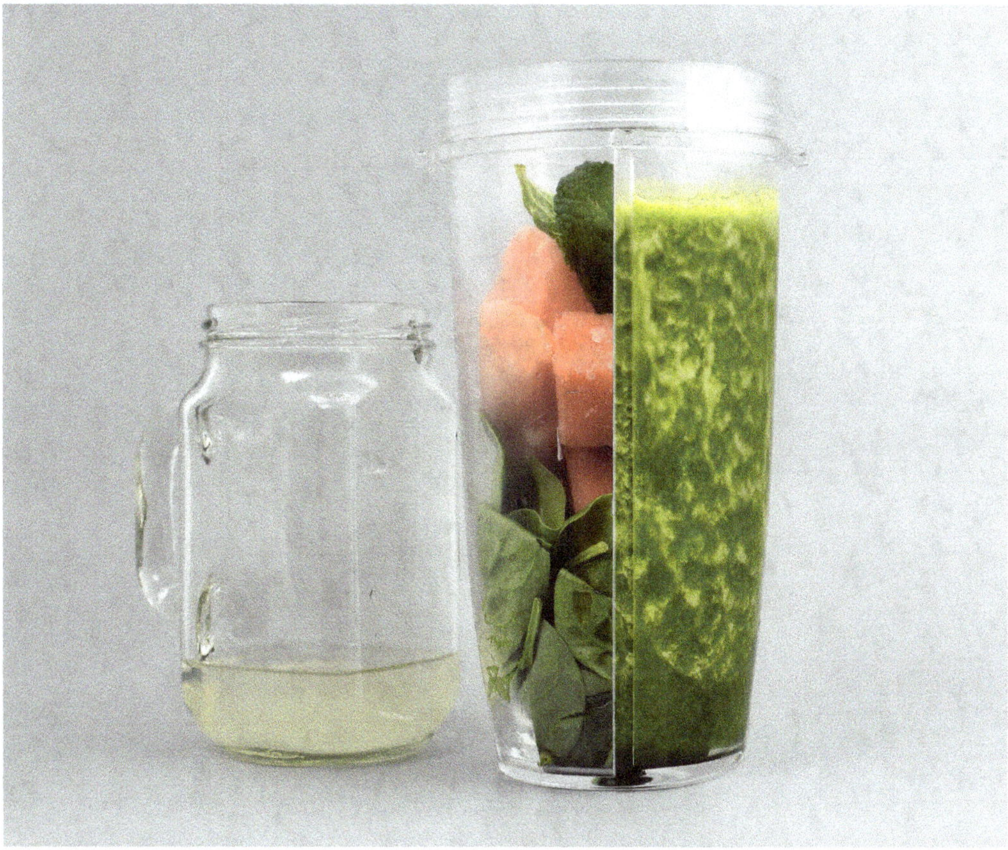

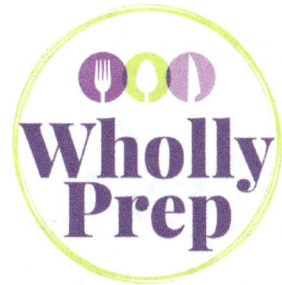

Place **greens**, chopped **watermelon**, and **mint** in a freezer-safe container and freeze up to 3 months.

To prepare smoothie, dump all frozen ingredients into a blender, add **water and citrus juice,** and puree until smooth.

PB CHOCOLATE AMOR

INGREDIENTS

2 handfuls greens
2 frozen bananas
2 Tbsp peanut butter
2 Tbsp cocoa powder
1 Tbsp flaxseed meal
1 cup non-dairy milk

Wholly Prep

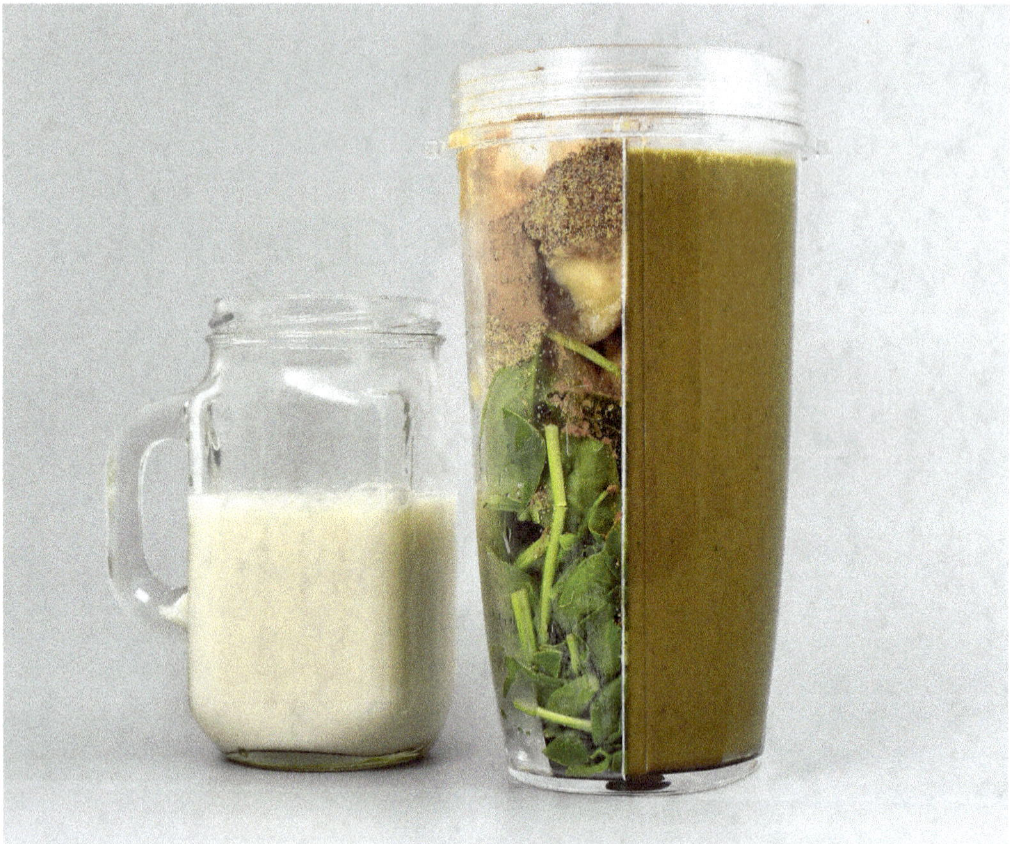

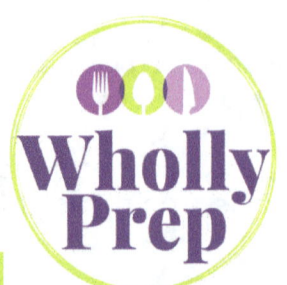

Place **greens**, **flax meal**, **cocoa powder**, **peanut butter**, and peeled, sliced **bananas** in a freezer-safe container and freeze up to 3 months.

To prepare smoothie, dump all frozen ingredients into a blender, add **non-dairy milk.** and puree until smooth.

PEACH MANGO

INGREDIENTS

2 handfuls greens
1 cup frozen mango
1 cup frozen peaches
1 Tbsp flaxseed meal
1 cup water

Wholly Prep

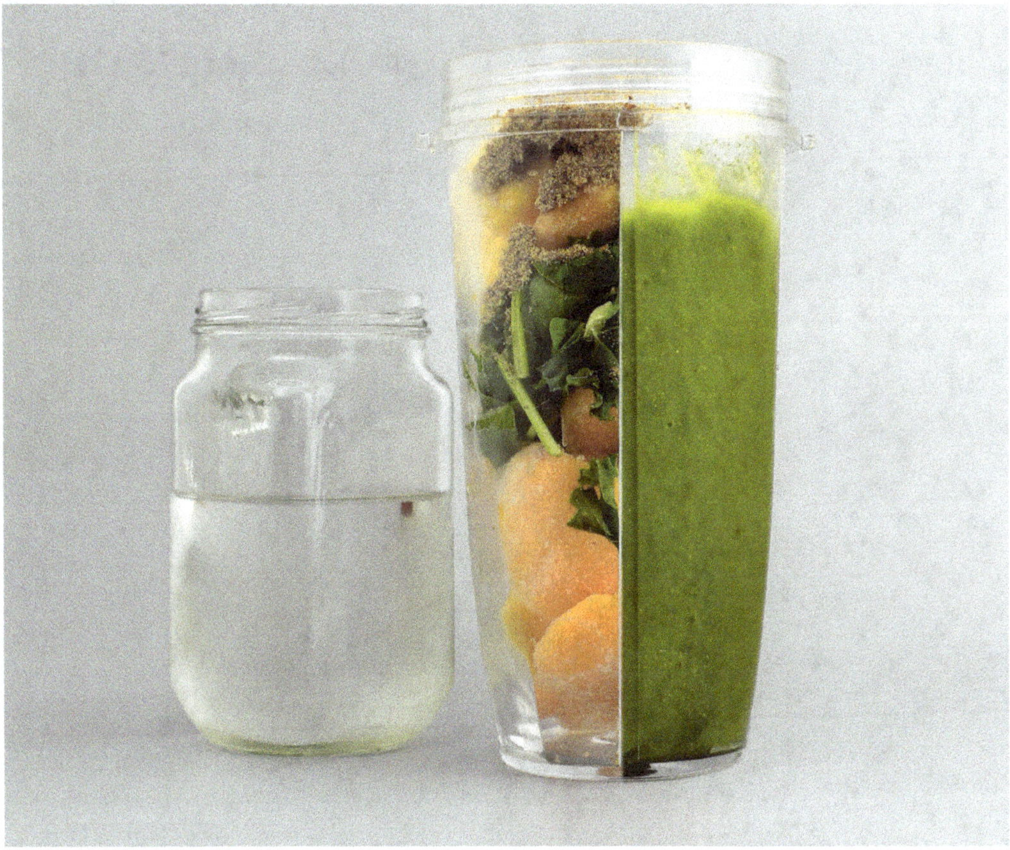

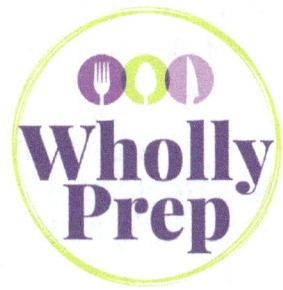

Place **greens**, chopped **mango** and **peaches**, and **flaxseed meal** in a freezer-safe container and freeze up to 3 months.

To prepare smoothie, dump all frozen ingredients into a blender, add **water,** and puree until smooth.

PICK-ME-UP

INGREDIENTS

2 handfuls spinach
½ frozen avocado
¼ cup espresso or concentrated brewed coffee
¾ cup non-dairy milk
1 tsp cinnamon
2 dates, pitted
1 Tbsp flaxseed meal
1 tsp maca powder (optional)

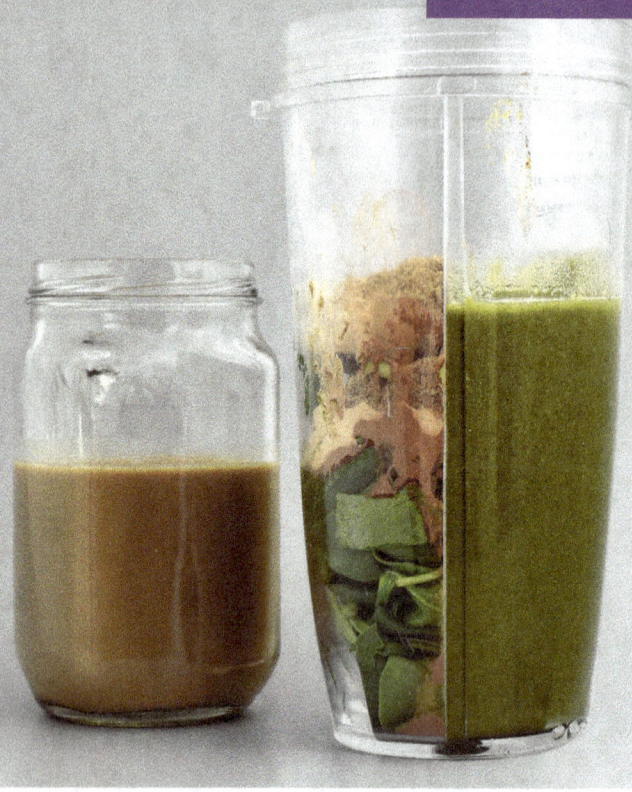

Time-Saving Tip: Brew strong cold-pressed coffee overnight in a French press.

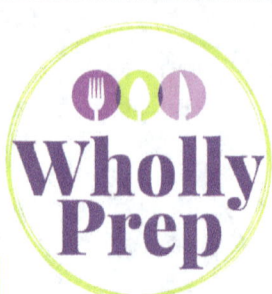

Place **spinach**, pitted **avocado** and **dates**, **flaxseed meal**, **maca powder**, and **cinnamon** in a freezer-safe container and freeze up to 3 months.

To prepare smoothie, dump all frozen ingredients into a blender and add **non-dairy milk**. Brew **strong coffee** and add 1/4 cup to blender and puree until smooth.

PISTACHIO COCONUT

INGREDIENTS

2 handfuls spinach
1 cup coconut milk
1 frozen banana
½ cup shelled, unsalted pistachios
2 Tbsp coconut flakes

Tip: Blend the coconut flakes in the smoothie or garnish with them, depending on texture preferences. Garnish with extra crushed pistachios, if desired.

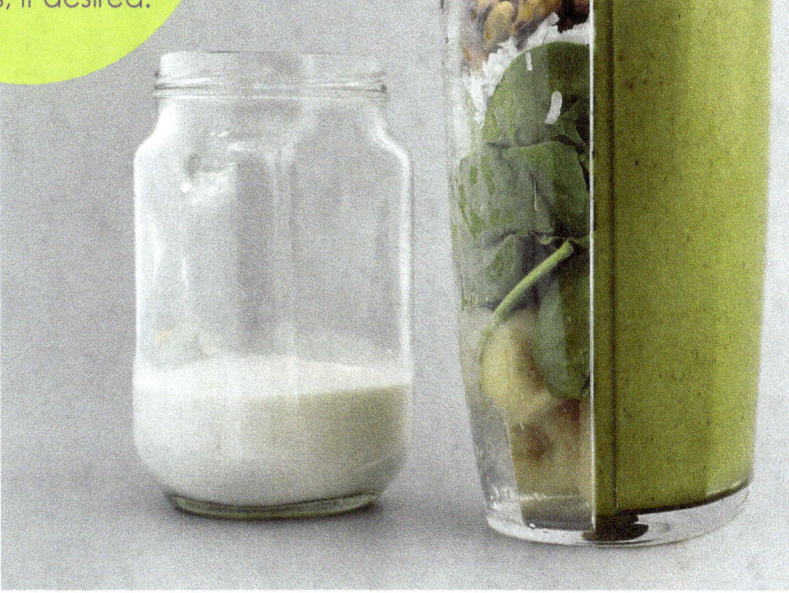

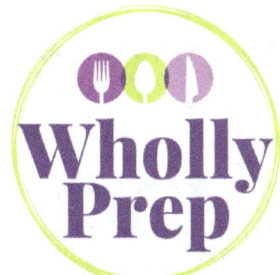

Place **spinach**, shelled **pistachios**, **coconut flakes**, and peeled, sliced **banana** in a freezer-safe container and freeze up to 3 months.

To prepare smoothie, dump all frozen ingredients into a blender, add **coconut milk**, and puree until smooth.

STRAWBERRY MANGO 'N' GREENS

INGREDIENTS

2 handfuls greens
1 cup frozen strawberries
1 cup frozen mango chunks
1 Tbsp chia seeds
1 cup non-dairy milk
1 sweet apple, cored and sliced (Pink lady, Honeycrisp)

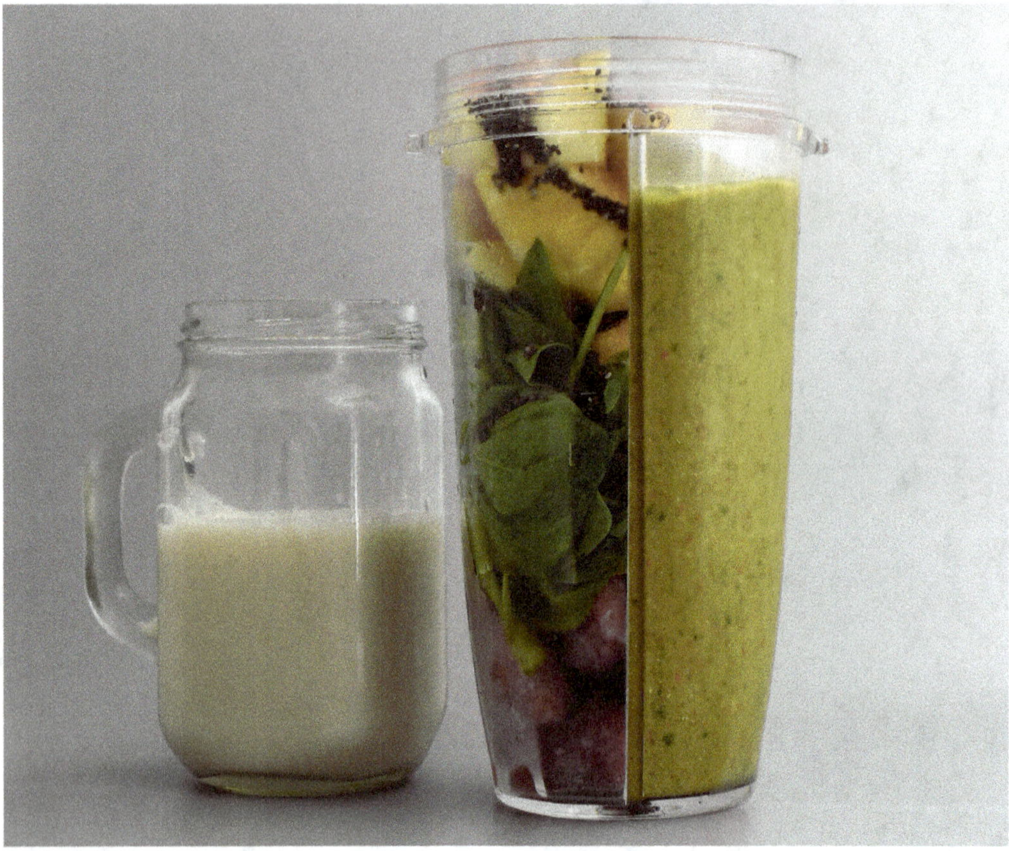

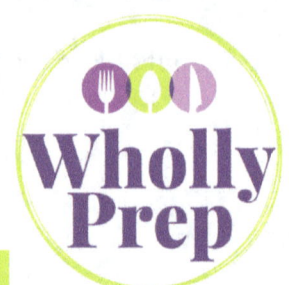

Place **greens**, **mango chunks**, **chia seeds**, **strawberries**, and cored, sliced **apple** in a freezer-safe container and freeze up to 3 months.

To prepare smoothie, dump all frozen ingredients into a blender, add **non-dairy milk**, and puree until smooth.

SUPERFOODS

☆☆☆☆☆

INGREDIENTS

2 handfuls kale
1 cup almond milk
2 frozen kiwis, peeled
½ cup frozen mixed berries
1/2 frozen banana
2 dates, pitted
10 mint leaves
1/2 tsp spirulina powder
1 Tbsp chia seeds

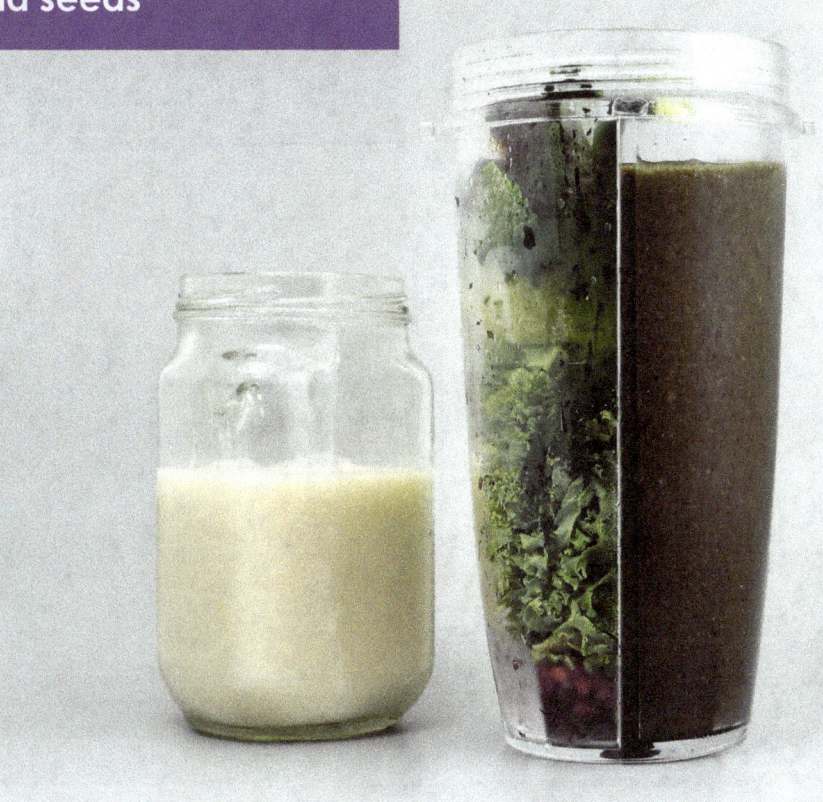

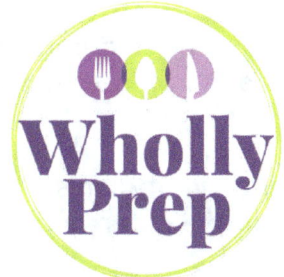

Place **kale**, peeled **kiwis**, pitted **dates**, **chia seeds**, **spirulina powder**, **mixed berries**, **mint**, and peeled, sliced **banana** in a freezer-safe container and freeze up to 3 months.

To prepare smoothie, dump all frozen ingredients into a blender, add **almond milk,** and puree until smooth.

THE CURE

☆☆☆☆☆

INGREDIENTS

1 handful greens
½ cucumber, chopped
½ carrot, chopped
½ celery stalk, chopped
2 Roma tomatoes, seeded and chopped
¼ cup parsley
¾ cup water
1 tsp soy sauce
1 tsp apple cider vinegar
handful of ice

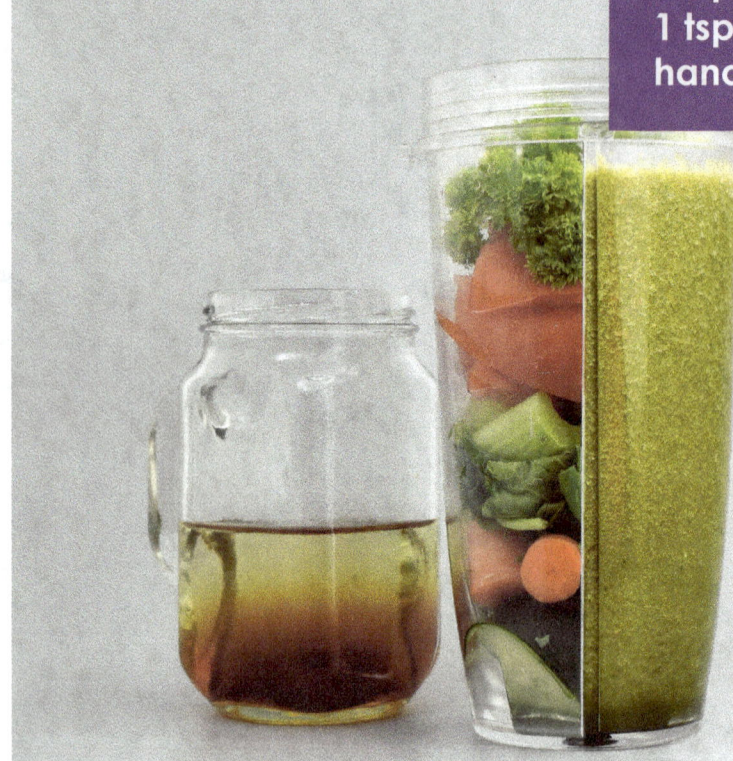

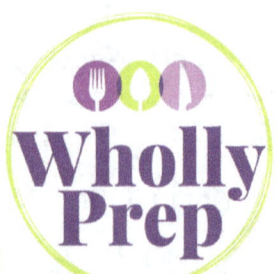

Place **greens**, **parsley**, chopped **cucumber**, **celery**, and **carrots**, and seeded **Roma tomatoes** in a freezer-safe container and freeze up to 3 months.

To prepare smoothie, dump all frozen ingredients into a blender, add **water, soy sauce, apple cider vinegar, and ice,** and puree until smooth.

THE ZINGER

INGREDIENTS

2 handfuls greens
1 cup non-dairy milk
1 frozen banana
1 avocado
1 sweet sliced apple (Pink Lady or Honeycrisp)
1 inch fresh peeled ginger
6 inches celery stalk
3 dates, pitted

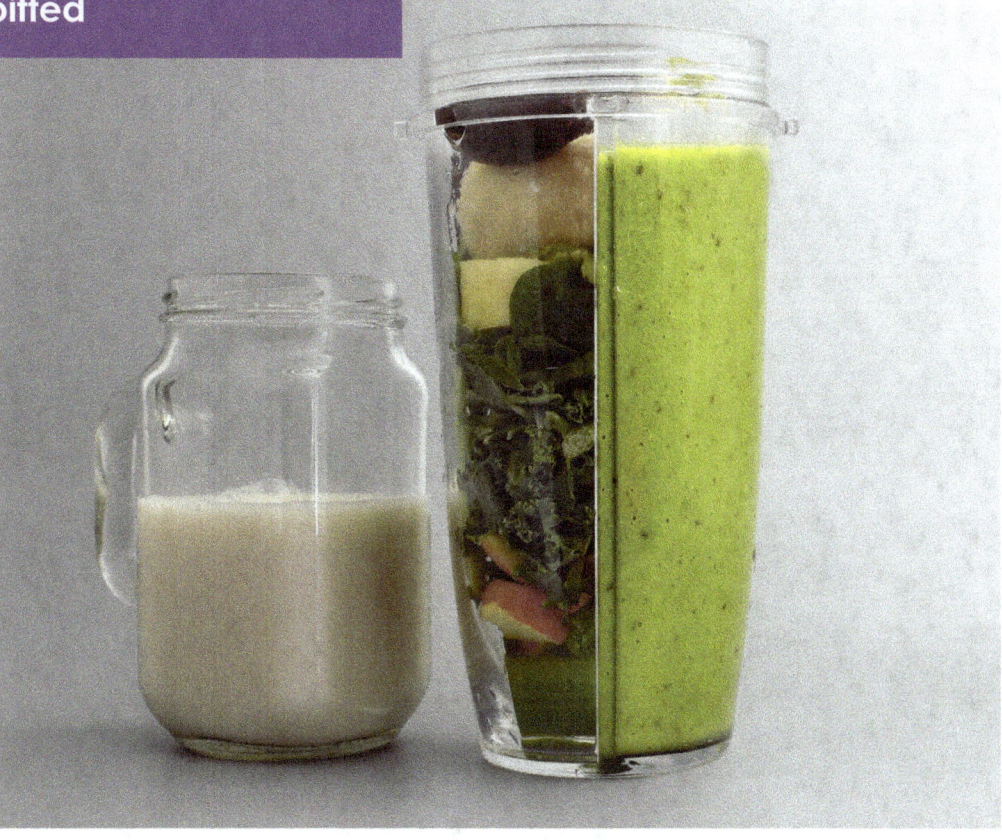

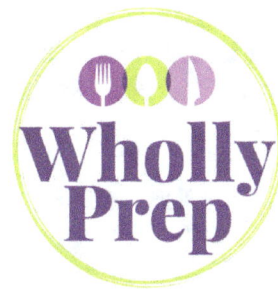

Place **greens**, pitted **avocado** and **dates**, chopped **celery**, peeled **ginger**, cored and chopped **apple**, and peeled, sliced **banana** in a freezer-safe container and freeze up to 3 months.

To prepare smoothie, dump all frozen ingredients into a blender, add **non-dairy milk,** and puree until smooth.

TROPICAL GREEN SMOOTHIE

☆☆☆☆☆

INGREDIENTS

2 handfuls of greens
1 frozen banana
½ cup frozen mango chunks
½ cup frozen pineapple chunks
1 Tbsp hemp seeds
3/4 cup water

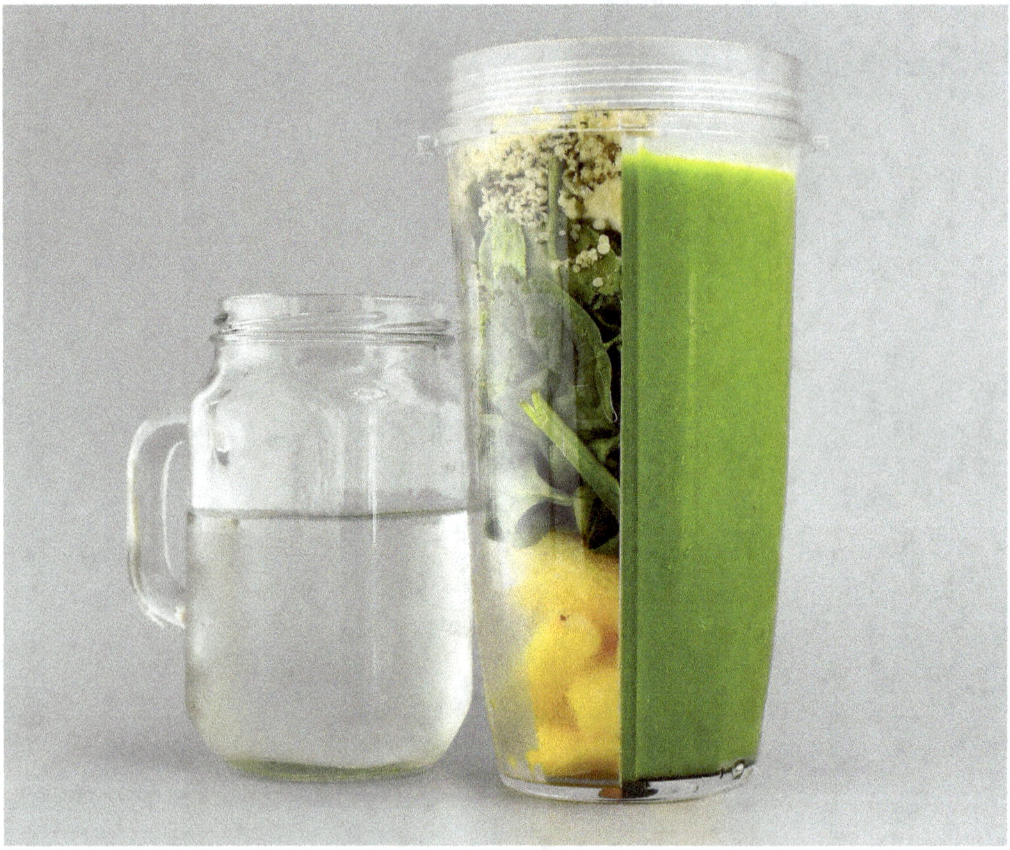

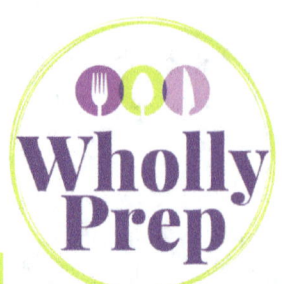

Place **greens**, **hemp seeds**, **mango chunks**, **pineapple chunks**, and peeled, sliced **banana** in a freezer-safe container and freeze up to 3 months.

To prepare smoothie, dump all frozen ingredients into a blender, add **water**, and puree until smooth.

REFERENCES & RESOURCES

Measurements & Conversions

Cup to Tablespoon to Teaspoon to Milliliters
1 cup = 16 Tbsp = 48 tsp = 240 ml
¾ cup = 12 Tbsp = 36 tsp = 180 ml
½ cup = 8 Tbsp = 24 tsp = 120 ml
¼ cup = 4 Tbsp = 12 tsp = 60 ml
1 Tbsp = 3 tsp = 15 ml
1 tsp = 5 ml

Cup to Fluid Ounces
1 cup = 8 fl oz
3/4 cup = 6 fl oz
2/3 cup = 5 fl oz
1/2 cup = 4 fl oz
1/3 cup = 3 fl oz
1/4 cup = 2 fl oz

Index

A

almond butter 14, 21
apple 33, 40, 42, 43
apple cider vinegar 42
avocado 15, 21

B

banana 14, 15, 16, 17, 21, 24, 27, 28, 29, 30, 32, 33, 34, 36, 39, 41, 43, 44
blender 12

C

cantaloupe 15
celery 26, 42, 43
cherry 19, 23
chia seeds 16, 18, 19, 21, 31, 40, 41
chocolate 34
cilantro 20
cinnamon 24, 38
cocoa powder 21, 22, 36
coconut flakes 29, 39
coffee 38
cucumber 20, 26, 42

D

date 11, 15, 18, 21, 22, 24, 28, 32, 38, 41, 43

F

flaxseed meal 17, 24, 30, 33, 36, 37, 38

G

ginger 25, 43
grape 26

H

hemp seed 7, 14, 15, 34, 44
honeydew 15

J

jalapeño 20

K

kale 10, 11, 26, 41
kiwi 26, 41

L

lemon juice 35
lime 19, 20

M

maca 7, 38
mandarin 16
mango 37, 40, 44
mint 20, 34, 35, 41
mixed berries 17, 18, 41

O

oats 24, 28, 32
orange 27, 31

P

parsley 42
peach 19, 25, 32, 37
peanut butter 17, 28, 36
pear 14
pineapple 29, 31, 44
pistachios 39
plant-based diet 7, 8, 9, 49

S

soy sauce 42
spinach 7, 10, 11, 17, 23, 24, 25, 27, 28, 33, 38, 39
spirulina 41
strawberry 18, 22, 28, 33, 40

T

tomato 42

V

vanilla 18, 21, 22, 23, 24, 27

W

watermelon 35
Wholly Prep 9

About the Author

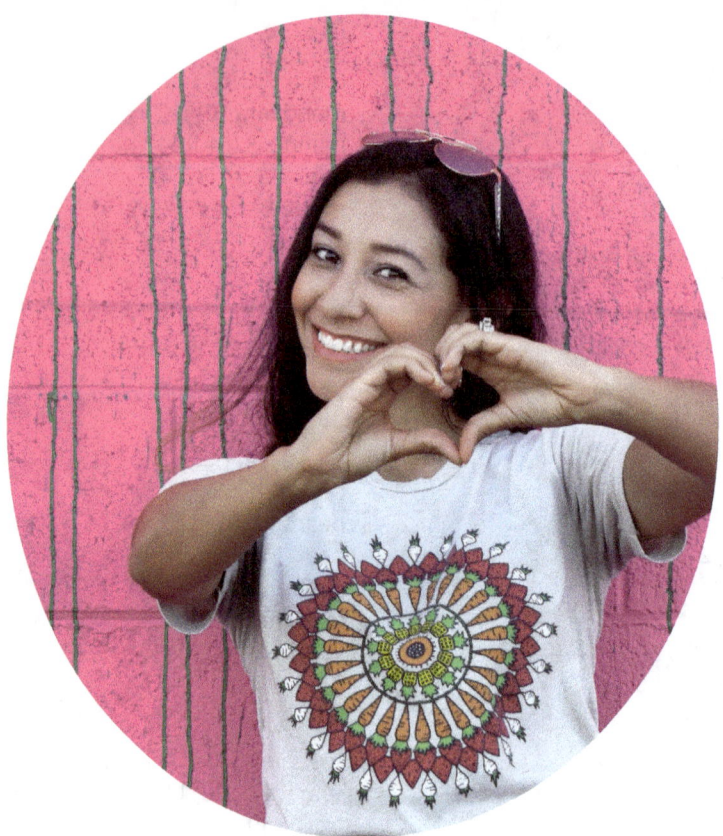

Farin Montañez is an ultramarathon runner, a mother of two, and a military wife who lives in Central California. She holds a B.A. in Mass Communication and Journalism from Fresno State and is a Certified Holistic Nutritionist.

Farin blogs about nutrition, running, and productivity — and shares plant-based recipes — at SpiritedVegan.com.

She developed the Wholly Prep framework to make it easier for people to eat a whole food, plant-based diet while saving time in the kitchen and money at the grocery store.

Learn how to meal prep a week's worth of nutritious, disease-fighting meals in two hours at **SpiritedVegan.com/WhollyPrep** and look out for more Wholly Prep recipe books.

LET'S CONNECT!

facebook.com/spiritedvegan
instagram.com/spiritedvegan
twitter.com/spirited_vegan
spiritedvegan.com

www.ingramcontent.com/pod-product-compliance
Lightning Source LLC
Chambersburg PA
CBHW051354070526
44584CB00025B/3762